Obs̶ ̶ ̶ ̶ ̶ ̶ ̶ ̶ ̶ ̶ ̶ / in Primary Care

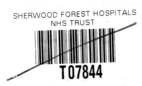

Manish Latthe, Sirjit S Bath, Pallavi M Latthe (Editors)

Dr Manish Latthe MA MBBS MRCGP DRCOG DFFP
General Practitioner/GP Trainer
Tower Hill Medical Centre, Great Barr, Birmingham
and
Associate Fellow, Centre for Primary Health Care Studies, University of Warwick

Dr Sirjit S Bath MBChB DGM DFFP
General Practitioner/GP Trainer/GP Tutor/PCT Board Member
Tower Hill Medical Centre, Great Barr, Birmingham

Dr Pallavi M Latthe MBBS MD MRCOG DFFP
Specialist Registrar in Obstetrics and Gynaecology/WellBeing
Research Fellow
Birmingham Women's Hospital, Edgbaston, Birmingham

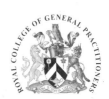

The Royal College of General Practitioners was founded in 1952 with this object:

"To encourage, foster and maintain the highest possible standards in general practice and for that purpose to take or join with others in taking steps consistent with the charitable nature of that object which may assist towards the same."

Among its responsibilities under its Royal Charter the College is entitled to:

"Diffuse information on all matters affecting general practice and issue such publications as may assist the object of the College."

British Library Cataloguing-in-Publication Data
A catalogue record for this book is available from the British Library

© Royal College of General Practitioners 2003
Published by the Royal College of General Practitioners 2003
14 Princes Gate, Hyde Park, London, SW7 1PU

Disclaimer
This publication is intended for the use of medical practitioners in the UK and not for patients. The authors, editors, and Publisher have taken care to ensure that the information contained in this book is correct to the best of their knowledge, at the time of publication. While efforts have been made to ensure the accuracy of the information presented, particularly that related to the prescription of drugs, the authors, editors, and Publisher cannot accept liability for information that is subsequently shown to be wrong. Readers are advised to check that the information, especially that related to drug usage, complies with information contained in the *British National Formulary*, or equivalent, or manufacturers' datasheets, and that it complies with the latest legislation and standards of practice.

Designed and typeset by Hobbs the Printers
Printed by Hobbs the Printers
Indexed by Dr Olivera Potparic

ISBN: 0 85084 285 9

Contents

Authors   v

Foreword   ix

Glossary   xi

Abnormalities of Menstruation   1

The Menopause and Hormone Replacement Therapy   19

Incontinence and Prolapse   35

Screening and Cancers in Gynaecology   57

Pelvic Infections and Vaginitis   69

Pelvic Pain   81

Subfertility   93

Family Planning   105

Routine Antenatal and Postnatal Care   119

Problems in Early Pregnancy   131

Problems in Later Pregnancy   143

Evidence-based Medicine in Obstetrics and Gynaecology   159

Index   167

Authors

ABNORMALITIES OF MENSTRUATION
Dr Manish Latthe (editor)

THE MENOPAUSE AND HORMONE REPLACEMENT THERAPY
Dr Manish Latthe (editor)

INCONTINENCE AND PROLAPSE
Mr Philip Tooz Hobson
Consultant Obstetrician and Urogynaecologist
Birmingham Women's Healthcare NHS Trust
Edgbaston
Birmingham

Dr Samantha Pretlove
Clinical Research Fellow
Department of Obstetrics and Gynaecology
2nd floor, Academic Library
Birmingham Women's Healthcare NHS Trust
Edgbaston
Birmingham

SCREENING AND CANCERS IN GYNAECOLOGY
Dr Pallavi M Latthe (editor)

Mr Mahmood Shafi
Consultant Gynaecological Oncologist
Birmingham Women's Healthcare NHS Trust
Edgbaston
Birmingham

Mr Santanu Baruah
Newtown Road
Worcester
Worcestershire

PELVIC INFECTIONS AND VAGINITIS
Dr Manish Latthe (editor)
Dr Pallavi M Latthe (editor)
Dr Sirjit S Bath (editor)

PELVIC PAIN
Dr Swati Jha
Obstetrics and Gynaecology
Dudley Group of Hospitals NHS Trust
Wordsley Hospital
Stream Road
Stourbridge
West Midlands

SUBFERTILITY
Dr Pallavi M Latthe (editor)

Mr Stephen Keay
Consultant Obstetrics and Gynaecology
Department of Obstetrics and Gynaecology
Walsgrave Hospitals NHS Trust
Clifford Bridge Road
Coventry

FAMILY PLANNING
Dr Rajvir Thandi
Northbrook Group Practice
93 Northbrook Road
Shirley
Solihull
West Midlands

Dr Wendy Milligan
Northbrook Group Practice
93 Northbrook Road
Shirley
Solihull
West Midlands

ROUTINE ANTENATAL AND POSTNATAL CARE
Dr Sirjit S Bath (editor)
Dr Manish Latthe (editor)

PROBLEMS IN EARLY PREGNANCY
Dr Sirjit S Bath (editor)
Dr Manish Latthe (editor)

PROBLEMS IN LATER PREGNANCY
Dr Arri Coomarasamy MBChB MRCOG
Specialist Registrar in Obstetrics and Gynaecology and Honorary Lecturer in Public
Health and Epidemiology
Birmingham Women's Hospital
Metchley Park Road
Edgbaston
Birmingham

Dr D van der Berg DRCOG
General Practice Registrar
57 Woodland Road
Northfield
Birmingham

EVIDENCE-BASED MEDICINE IN OBSTETRICS AND GYNAECOLOGY
Dr Arri Coomarasamy MBChB MRCOG
Specialist Registrar in Obstetrics and Gynaecology and Honorary Lecturer in Public
Health and Epidemiology
Birmingham Women's Hospital
Metchley Park Road
Edgbaston
Birmingham

The editors would like to thank the following for their support in producing the book:

Dr Rodger Charlton, Helen Farrelly and Patrick O'Brien at the RCGP, and Dr Debal Nandi and Dr V Sandra Calderwood at Tower Hill Medical Centre

Foreword

Of not many books can a doctor in primary care honestly say, "What a relief to have this on the consulting room bookshelf" – but the present volume is assuredly one of them.

It is still not all that long since the caricature of the GP was someone who could largely conceal out-of-date knowledge and skills behind a good bedside manner and a low threshold for specialist referral. Recent years have seen a welcome revolution in what is expected of general practice, not least by us, its practitioners. The GP of the new century is proud and relieved to be offered the rewarding chance – indeed, the incentive – to provide high-quality diagnosis and to undertake management and treatments once the province of secondary care.

Obstetrics and gynaecology are 'high profile' subjects in general practice. Seeing a woman through pregnancy and childbirth remains one of the most joyful episodes of long-term patient care, even if intrapartum care is no longer the norm. And dealing competently with gynaecological problems makes an invaluable contribution to the well-being not just of the patient but of her partner(s) and family too.

In both areas, safety of course remains paramount. The best safeguard continues to be a sound foundation in up-to-date evidence-based knowledge and a sense of satisfaction in maintaining clinical skills – exactly what this title provides.

Obstetrics and Gynaecology in Primary Care is a comprehensive source-book that will benefit both the doctor who regularly refers to it and, more importantly, his or her patients. It has been painstakingly collated by experienced and enthusiastic GPs and colleagues and is, above all, eminently practical in its approach. You will find, for example, guidance on taking difficult cervical smears, advice on patients late for their depot contraception, and selected website addresses included among the references.

I congratulate the authors most warmly, and can pay them no greater tribute than to say how much I wish their book had been available earlier in my own career.

Roger Neighbour
President of the Royal College of General Practitioners
GP, formerly of Abbots Langley, Hertfordshire
Author of *The Inner Consultation* and *The Inner Apprentice*

Glossary

ACE	angiotensin-converting enzyme
ADH	antidiuretic hormone
AFP	alpha-foetoprotein
AIS	adenocarcinoma in-situ
APH	antepartum haemorrhage
ARC	antenatal results and choices
b–hCG	free beta-subunit of human chorionic gonadotrophin
BMI	body mass index
BNA	borderline nuclear abnormality
BNF	British National Formulary
BP	blood pressure
BRCA	breast cancer genes
CCF	congestive cardial failure
CDSR	Cochrane Database of Systematic Reviews
CEA	carcinoembryonic antigen
CGIN	cervical glandular intraepithelial neoplasia
CIN	cervical intraepithelial neoplasia
CINAHL	Cumulative Index to Nursing and Allied Health Literature
CISC	clean intermittent self-catheterisation
CMV	cytomegalovirus
CNS	central nervous system
COCP	combined oral contraceptive pill
CPP	chronic pelvic pain
CTG	cardiotocography
CVA	cerebrovascular accident
CVS	chorionic villus sampling
D+C	dilation and curettage
DARE	Database of Abstracts of Reviews of Effects
DEXA	dual energy X-ray absorptiometry
DFFP	Diploma of the Faculty of Family Planning and Reproductive Health Care

DHEAS	dihydroepiandrosterone sulfate
DoH	Department of Health
DUB	dysfunctional uterine bleeding
EBM	evidence-based medicine
EDD	estimated date of delivery
EPAU	early pregnancy assessment unit
ERPOC	evacuation of the retained products of conception
ESR	erythrocyte sedimentation rate
FBC	full blood count
FGR	foetal growth restriction
FPA	Family Planning Association
FSH	follicle-stimulating hormone
FTT	failure to thrive
GDM	gestational diabetes mellitus
GI	gastro-intestinal
GnRH	gonadotrophin-releasing hormone
GP	general practitioner
GUM	genito-urinary medicine
HbA1c	haemoglobin A1c test, glycosylated haemoglobin A1c test, glycohaemoglobin A1c test, or A1c test
hCG	human chorionic gonadotropin
HELLP	haemolysis, elevated liver enzymes, low platelets
HERS	Heart and Estrogen/progestin Replacement Study
HFEA	Human Fertilisation and Embryology Authority
HIV	human immunodeficiency virus
HPV	human papillomavirus
HRT	hormone replacement therapy
HSIL	high-grade squamous intraepithelial lesion
HSV	herpes simplex virus
ICS	International Continence Society (UK)
ICSI	intracytoplasmic sperm injection
IU(C)D	intrauterine (contraceptive) device
IUGR	intrauterine growth restriction
IUI	intrauterine insemination
IUS	intrauterine system
IVF	in vitro fertilisation

LBC	liquid-based cytology
LH	luteinising hormone
LLETZ	large loop excision of transformation zone
LMP	last menstrual period
LSIL	low-grade squamous intraepithelial lesion
LUNA	laparoscopic uterosacral nerve ablation
MAOI	monoamine oxidase inhibitors
MI	myocardial infarction
MIMS	Monthly Index of Medical Specialities
MRC	Medical Research Council
MRI	magnetic resonance imaging
MS	multiple sclerosis
MSU	mid-stream urine
NHS	National Health Service
NHSCSP	NHS Cervical Screening Programme
NICE	National Institute for Clinical Excellence
NIDDM	non-insulin dependent diabetes mellitus
NLM	National Library of Medicine
NNT	number needed to treat
NSAIDs	non-steroidal anti-inflammatory drugs
NSC	National Screening Committee
NT	nuchal translucency
NTD	neural tube defect
PCC	post-coital contraception
PCG	primary care group
PCOS	polycystic ovarian syndrome
PCR	polymerise chain reaction
PCT	primary care team
PESA	percutaneous epididymal sperm aspiration
PFI	Pill-free interval
PHCT	primary health care team
PID	pelvic inflammatory disease
PMS	premenstrual syndrome
PPROM	pre-term pre-labour rupture of membranes
RCGP	Royal College of General Practitioners
RCOG	Royal College of Obstetricians and Gynaecologists
RCT	randomised controlled trial
Rh	Rhesus

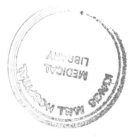

SCJ	squamo-columnar junction
SFA	seminal fluid analysis
SGA	small for gestational age
SHBG	sex hormone binding globulin
SIGN	Scottish Intercollegiate Guidelines Network
SR	systematic review
SSRIs	selective serotonin reuptake inhibitors
STD	sexually transmitted disease
STI	sexually transmitted infection
TAH	total abdominal hysterectomy
TCRE	transcervical resection of the endometrium
TENS	transcutaneous electrical nerve stimulation
TESA	testicular sperm aspiration
TORCH	a blood test that screens for several congenital infections, including toxoplasmosis, rubella, cytomegalovirus, herpes simplex, and other infections
TSH	thyroid-stimulating hormone
TVT	tension-free vaginal tape
UDCA	ursodeoxycholic acid
uE3	unconjugated oestriol
UPSI	unprotected sexual intercourse
USS	ultrasound scan
UTI	urinary tract infection
VaIN	vaginal intraepithelial neoplasia
VDRL	venereal disease research laboratory
VIN	vulval intraepithelial neoplasia
VTE	venous thromboembolism
WHI	Woman's Health Initiative
WHO	World Health Organization

Abnormalities of Menstruation

Dr Manish Latthe

Introduction

Disorders of menstruation are among the commonest gynaecological presenting complaints to GPs, and the leading cause of referral to hospital gynaecologists. These disorders can have a major effect upon sufferers' social and psychological well-being as well as their physical health. In order to treat these disorders, it is useful first to consider the normal menstrual cycle.

The Menstrual Cycle

Menstruation is the cyclic monthly bloody vaginal discharge of sloughed-off endometrium. It occurs throughout a woman's reproductive life. The onset of menstruation is known as menarche. Menopause, on the other hand, is the stage at which ovaries stop producing eggs, menstrual activity decreases and eventually ceases, and the body decreases the production of the female hormones, oestrogen and progesterone.

The first day of menses is day 1 of the menstrual cycle. The average duration of menses is five ($\pm$ 2) days; the median length of the cycle is 28 days, but ranges from 25–36 days for ovulatory cycles. The usual range of blood loss per cycle is 40–79ml, with menorrhagia considered present if blood loss is 80ml or higher. Menstrual blood does not normally clot unless bleeding is very heavy. A typical saturated pad or tampon absorbs between 20–30ml.

The menstrual cycle can be divided into three phases. The follicular phase extends from the first day of menses to the day before the preovulatory LH surge. Its length is the most variable of the phases. The ovulatory phase is a series of complex endocrine events that culminates in the LH surge. As LH and progesterone levels increase, oestradiol levels decrease. The LH surge usually lasts 36–48 hours and consists of multiple large bursts of LH released in pulses. The LH surge, which results in complete maturation of the follicle, is necessary for ovulation (i.e. release of the ovum from the mature Graafian follicle), which usually occurs 16–32 hours after onset of the surge.

The luteal phase follows, and the length of this phase is the most constant, averaging 14 days and ending with day 1 of the cycle. The length corresponds to the functional life span of the corpus luteum, which secretes progesterone and oestradiol for about 14 days, then degenerates unless pregnancy ensues. Implantation of a fertilised ovum is supported by the corpus luteum (by secreting progesterone in increasing quantities peaking six to eight days after the LH surge). Progesterone causes the basal body temperature to increase by 0.5°C during the luteal phase and the level remains elevated until menstruation.

If fertilisation occurs, HCG from the fertilised ovum supports the corpus luteum until the foeto-placental unit can support itself. During most of the luteal phase, circulating LH and FSH levels decrease and are low, but they begin to increase with menstruation in the following cycle.

Premenstrual Syndrome

Premenstrual syndrome (sometimes called premenstrual tension) is a disorder defined by features including 'non-specific somatic, psychological or behavioural symptoms recurring in the premenstrual phase of the menstrual cycle' (O'Brien, 1987). The symptoms should be of sufficient severity to produce social, family, or occupational disruption, and have occurred in at least four of the previous six cycles, typically some seven to ten days before menses and lasting until a few hours after menses start. Possibly as many as 75% of menstruating women have some premenstrual symptoms.

Causes
- PMS appears to be related to cyclic changes in the levels of the female hormones, oestrogen and progesterone. Symptoms of PMS change with hormonal manipulations and disappear with pregnancy and menopause.
- Chemical changes in the brain may also be involved; it is thought that fluctuations of serotonin are an important factor, especially in cases of depression.

Diagnosis
A careful history will pinpoint the diagnosis in the majority of cases. The type and intensity of symptoms will vary in each patient and from cycle to cycle. In some women, symptoms are significant but brief and not disabling; in others, normal functioning is disturbed. Symptoms can last from a few hours to up to ten days.

The most common complaints are psychological, such as mood changes, irritability, nervousness, lack of control, agitation, anger, insomnia, difficulty in concentrating, lethargy, depression, and fatigue. Oedema, breast fullness, and pain can occur. In addition, headache, vertigo, syncope, paraesthesiae of the extremities, easy bruising, and cardiac palpitation can occur. Other symptoms include constipation, nausea, vomiting, and changes in appetite, and pelvic heaviness or pressure and backache may occur. Aggravation of some skin disorders such as acne may also occur.

Treatment

Counselling may be useful to help the woman and her family cope with PMS. The woman's activities should be modified to reduce stress.

Exercise is helpful for PMS because it reduces stress and tension, acts as a mood elevator, provides a sense of well-being, and improves blood circulation by increasing the natural production of beta-endorphins. Exercise should be at least three times weekly for 20–30 minutes each time.

Dietary advice includes eating smaller meals more frequently, ensuring that they are high in complex carbohydrates and low in simple sugars. This helps to maintain a steady blood glucose level. Patients may also benefit from reducing their intake of caffeine, alcohol, salt, and fat.

Some doctors suggest that supplemental vitamins and minerals may be taken to relieve some PMS symptoms, particularly vitamin B6 (orally 100mg daily from day 10 of one cycle to day 3 of the next cycle), B complex, vitamin E, and vitamin C. Of these, only vitamin B6 has any evidence to support its effectiveness. However, both oral magnesium (200mg daily) and calcium (1200mg daily) have been shown to be beneficial. Evening primrose oil (40mg orally up to eight times daily) has some evidence showing it to be effective for treating the psychological symptoms. The fruit extract agnus castus has also been shown to be effective in reducing PMS symptoms (dry extract tablets, one tablet daily).

Fluid retention can be treated using a diuretic (e.g. hydrochlorothiazide 25–50mg per day orally), starting just before symptoms are expected.

Use of the COCP is an effective treatment, as it suppresses ovulation and the associated cyclical changes, and is especially useful in women who require contraception as well.

The use of progestogens in PMS is controversial. Progestogens can be given by various routes – including vaginal gel, suppository, intra-muscular injection (e.g. medroxyprogesterone acetate, Depo-Provera®), oral progesterone tablets – taken for 10–14 days before the beginning of the period. The levonorgestrel-releasing intrauterine system (Mirena®) can improve symptoms of PMS in some women.

Selective serotonin reuptake inhibitors, such as fluoxetine 20mg daily and sertraline 50mg daily, are very effective drugs in the management of the psychological symptoms of PMS. Anxiolytics such as benzodiazepines have been used for irritability, nervousness, and lack of control. However, these are less suitable treatments because of their side-effects, especially dependency in long-term use.

Indications for referral to a gynaecologist
Referral to a specialist is rarely required but is warranted if the therapies tried in primary care are ineffective or if an underlying pathology is possibly present.

Secondary care treatments
- GnRH analogues (e.g. goserelin 3.6mg subcutaneously monthly) with low-dose oestrogen-progestogen 'add-back' therapy can be used in resistant cases.
- Levonorgestrel-releasing intrauterine system (Mirena®) with or without oestradiol implant or skin patches.
- Hysterectomy with bilateral salpingoophorectomy (as a last resort).

Useful tips
- By asking the woman to keep a symptom diary for two to three cycles, it is easier to confirm the diagnosis.
- Have a sympathetic attitude, explain the diagnosis, and reassure the patient that treatment is available, though most of the treatments are empirical.
- Emphasise lifestyle modifications, such as dietary changes and exercise, as this is also important to improve quality of life for sufferers.

Menorrhagia
Menorrhagia (heavy periods) is a major healthcare problem in the UK; 5% of women of reproductive age will seek help for this symptom annually. This group will have a lifetime risk of hysterectomy (primarily for menstrual disorders) of about 20%.

It is important to take a detailed history to establish if menorrhagia is present. The average volume of blood loss during menstruation is 40ml. Menorrhagia is objectively defined as a menstrual loss of over 80ml per month. Many women consider their menstruation to be excessive, but this amount of loss is actually present in about 10% of the population. For practical purposes, menorrhagia is defined as excessive menstrual blood loss interfering with the social and/or personal life of the woman.

Causes
- Menorrhagia can be associated with both ovulatory and anovulatory cycles. Ovulatory ovarian cycles give rise to regular menstrual cycles whereas anovulatory cycles result in irregular menstruation. Excessive menstrual loss in regular menstrual cycles is the commonest clinical presentation.
- Excessive menstrual loss in the absence of organic disease of the genital tract is known as dysfunctional uterine bleeding.
- Gynaecological pathology that can be associated with menorrhagia are fibroids, adenomyosis, PID, and endometrial hyperplasia.
- Hypothyroidism and disorders of haemostasis are rare causes of menorrhagia.

Investigations in primary care

Investigations should have three aims: to assess the morbidity associated with menorrhagia, to exclude major intrauterine disease, and to assess the role of coexistent disorders. These can be achieved through:

- *FBC.* Haemoglobin levels give an approximate assessment of the severity of losses (other indices of iron levels should also be considered).
- *Coagulation screen.* If specifically indicated from the history.
- *Thyroid function tests.* If specifically indicated from the history.
- *Other endocrine investigations.* There is no indication for any other endocrine investigations such as LH, FSH, or progesterone.

Investigations in secondary care

If your patient is referred to secondary care for further assessment, they may require other investigations:

- *Pelvic ultrasound.* It is of value in evaluating other pelvic disorders discovered during clinical examination.
- *Endometrial sampling.* This is combined with further assessment of the endometrial cavity; for example, hysteroscopy. This is done promptly in women over 40 years of age with intermenstrual bleeding, and after a failed trial of medical treatment.

Treatment of menorrhagia in primary care

As always, patient preference should be taken into account. The presence of ovulatory or anovulatory cycles is also an important consideration, as is the need for contraception.

In the management of excessive menstrual loss, many doctors do not necessarily prescribe the most effective treatments. In the UK, many GPs prescribe norethisterone, possibly the least effective option as first-line treatment, whereas tranexamic acid, probably the most effective first-line treatment, is prescribed much less often.

The aim of treatment is to reduce menstrual bleeding and thereby improve the quality of life. Further, treatment should aim to correct and prevent iron deficiency anaemia.

Non-hormonal treatments

- Tranexamic acid reduces menstrual loss by about 50–70%, when given in doses of 1–1.5g qds orally.
- NSAIDs reduce menstrual loss by about a third. They work by inhibiting prostaglandin synthetase. Mefenamic acid is the most widely used; the usual dose is 500mg tds orally.

Both of these non-hormonal therapies have the advantage of being taken only during menstruation itself – an aid to compliance – and are particularly useful in those women who either do not require contraception or do not wish to use a hormonal therapy. They are also of value in treating excessive menstrual blood loss associated with the use of non-hormonal IUCDs.

Hormonal treatments
- *Progestogens.* An example regime is norethisterone orally 5mg tds from day 5–25. Such treatments are now considered to be less effective but are still widely used in primary care (and even secondary care). Progestogens when given from day 19–26 are usually not effective.
- *COCP.* The combined contraceptive pill is a useful option, as it is both an effective contraceptive and treatment for menorrhagia. Like cyclical progestogens, COCPs are useful for anovulatory bleeding, as they provide a hormonal cycle.
- *Levonorgestrel-releasing intrauterine system (Mirena®).* This system consists of a T-shaped intrauterine device sheathed with a reservoir of levonorgestrel that is released at the rate of 20µg daily. This minimises the systemic progestogenic side-effects. As a result, patients are more likely to continue with this therapy than cyclical progestogen therapy. The commonest side-effect is irregular bleeding or spotting, especially in the first three months but which may occur for up to six months. However, by 12 months most women have only light bleeding and many are amenorrhoeic. Hence, pre-treatment counselling is very important to avoid discontinuation of the treatment by patients. The levonorgestrel-releasing intrauterine system is advocated as an alternative to surgery but whether this will provide a long-term alternative to surgery remains to be seen; initial studies indicate that it will help to reduce surgical intervention. It is also a useful treatment for dysmenorrhoea and PMS, and for when contraception is also required. The lifespan of the coil is five years and it is now licensed for treatment for menorrhagia.

Effective medical treatments exist and have a rational basis for their use. Increased use of effective treatments will improve patient choice and provide an alternative to surgery. Other treatments such as Danazol or GnRH analogues also work but should not be used as first-line therapy because of cost and side-effects.

Indications for referral to a gynaecologist or for surgical management
- Age over 40 years
- Associated problems like intermenstrual bleeding, dysmenorrhoea, or abnormal cervical smear
- Failed medical treatment
- Significant or persistent anaemia
- Abnormal gynaecological examination; e.g. bulky uterus

Figure 1.1: Medical management of the complaint of menorrhagia

```
                          ┌──────────────────────────────────┐
                          │ Does not require contraception or │
                          │ prefers non-hormonal treatment.   │
                          └──────────────────────────────────┘
```

| Mefenamic acid 500mg tds starting on first day of period for days of heavy flow (A). | Tranexamic acid 1g tds starting on first day of period for days of heavy flow (A). |

```
                          ┌──────────────────────────────────┐
                          │        Use for 3 months.         │
                          └──────────────────────────────────┘
```

| If blood flow is reduced to an acceptable level and no side effects treatment can continue indefinitely. | If blood flow not reduced to an acceptable level, or unacceptable side effects, try the other drug whilst awaiting REFERRAL. |

2   **3**

| Has copper or non-hormonal IUD in situ. | Needs contraception as well. |

| Add tranexamic acid or mefenamic acid (dosage as above) (A). | Change to progestogen-releasing IUD (A). | Combined oral contraceptive pill (A). | Progestogen-releasing IUD (A). | Long-acting progestogens (C). |

| If flow still unacceptable REMOVE IUD and suggest alternative contraception. | Review after **3 months**. Add mefenamic acid if necessary. | Review after **6 months**. If flow still unacceptable REFER. |

Review after **3 months**. If flow still unacceptable REFER.

| **While oral luteal phase progestogens are ineffective in reducing menstrual blood loss (A), intrauterine progestogens are effective (A).** |

Key: Grade A – based on RCTs; Grade C – based on more limited evidence but the advice relies on expert opinion and has the endorsement of respected authorities.
In: Royal College of Obstetricians and Gynaecologists. *The Initial Management of Menorrhagia. Evidence-based Guidelines No. 1.* London: RCOG Press, 1998; p10. © RCOG

Secondary care treatments
- Treatment of underlying causes; e.g. fibroids or endometriosis
- Endometrial ablation by various methods, such as TCRE or endometrial balloon ablation
- Hysterectomy, if conservative medical and surgical treatments have failed or have been declined, or there is associated pathology such as fibroids or atypical endometrial hyperplasia

---

Useful tips
- Before treating menorrhagia, exclude any underlying pathology by history, examination, and investigations.
- If a patient believes she has menorrhagia then she should be given treatment if she requests it.

Dysfunctional Uterine Bleeding
This is the commonest cause of abnormal vaginal bleeding. The diagnosis of DUB should be used only when other organic and structural causes for abnormal vaginal bleeding have been ruled out. It is most common at the extreme ages of a woman's reproductive years. Most severe cases of DUB occur in adolescent girls shortly after the onset of menstruation.

DUB may occur with anovulatory (>70% of episodes) or ovulatory cycles. The bleeding in anovulatory women (e.g. with polycystic ovaries) is caused by stimulation of the endometrium with unopposed oestrogen, which may result in endometrial hyperplasia. The endometrium sloughs incompletely and irregularly, and bleeding becomes irregular and sometimes excessive. In ovulatory cycles, abnormal bleeding is due to luteal phase irregularities.

History and physical examination cannot determine if endometrial hyperplasia is present. Those at higher risk of endometrial carcinoma should be referred for endometrial biopsy; i.e. women over 40 years of age, those with possible intrauterine disease (e.g. polyps), and those resistant to medical treatment.

Investigations in primary care
- FBC
- Cervical smear, if appropriate
- Pregnancy should be excluded by urinary pregnancy test
- Consider thyroid function tests, if appropriate
- Pelvic USS
- A menstrual calendar in which the patient keeps a detailed day-to-day record of the amount of loss for two to three months is useful to assess the severity and pattern of bleeding

Treatment in primary care

- Treat any underlying causes.
- Treatment of DUB varies with the age of the patient, the extent of the bleeding, pathologic assessment of the endometrium, and the patient's wishes.
- Oral iron therapy is often necessary to correct anaemia. Referral for blood transfusion is rarely required unless the patient is grossly anaemic.
- The first-line treatments are the same as for other causes of menorrhagia; i.e. tranexamic acid and mefenamic acid. Norethisterone (5mg tds orally from day 5 to day 26 of the cycle), COCPs, and the levonorgestrel-releasing intrauterine system are also recognised treatments.

Indications for referral to a gynaecologist

- Younger than age 11 (premenarchal)
- Abnormal bleeding accompanied by other symptoms
- Age over 40 years

Secondary care

Before instituting therapy, many gynaecologists perform endometrial sampling to diagnose intrauterine pathology and to exclude endometrial malignancy, particularly for at-risk patients; e.g. older than 40 years. Another option would be hysteroscopy and curettage.

Pelvic ultrasounds evaluate for fibroids or other structural lesions that may cause abnormal vaginal bleeding. Transvaginal ultrasound can be done when the patient may be pregnant, or may have anatomic problems or PCOS.

Useful tips

- The diagnosis of DUB is reached by exclusion of pelvic pathology.
- The assessment of severity and nature of DUB and wishes of the woman with respect to preservation of fertility or uterus and surgery can help with appropriate management.

Intermenstrual Bleeding

Intermenstrual bleeding – that is, vaginal bleeding between periods – is a distressing symptom for most women who suffer from this. While there are a number of underlying causes that need to be excluded, the commonest cause of abnormal vaginal bleeding during a woman's reproductive years is DUB, which is attributed to the fall in oestrogen secretion following ovulation.

Causes

- *Uterine.* Infection, DUB, endometrial polyps, submucosal fibroids, and endometrial cancer.

- *Cervical.* Cervicitis, cervical polyps, cervical intraepithelial neoplasia, or cervical cancer.
- *Vaginal.* Infection, injury from insertion of foreign objects, vaginal varicosities, malignancy.
- *Iatrogenic.* Irregular bleeding may occur as a side effect of combined and progestogen-only oral contraceptives, and other hormonal treatments. Medroxyprogesterone acetate (Depo-Provera®) can cause prolonged uterine breakthrough bleeding; this may continue after discontinuation of the drug because of persistent anovulation. The Norplant® system (surgically implanted levonorgestrel) has the same adverse effects as Depo-Provera®. Other drugs, such as anticoagulants, and use of an IUCD can occasionally cause intermenstrual bleeding.

Diagnosis

A thorough gynaecological history and examination is essential. The history must include age, parity, fertility, frequency, amount and pattern of bleeding in relation to the cycle, and the patient's plans with regard to contraception and future fertility. Any symptoms suggestive of hypothyroidism and bleeding disorder should be asked for as well as the drug history.

Abdominal and pelvic examination is essential. However, this may be deferred in young patients where there are no features suggestive of organic disease.

Investigations

- Genital swabs
- Cervical smear
- Thyroid function tests (if indicated)
- Coagulation screen (if indicated)

Management in primary care

- Treatment of genital infections such as bacterial vaginitis, Chlamydial cervicitis, etc as appropriate.
- Hormonal manipulation in cases of breakthrough bleeding on Depo-Provera®, COCPs, progestogen-only oral contraceptives, or the levonorgestrel-releasing intrauterine system. Usually, this is done by doubling the dose of the pills or commencing the combined oral contraceptive for two to three cycles.

Indications for referral to gynaecologist

- Abnormal cervical smear
- Cervical ectopy
- Suspicion of organic pathology such as polyps, fibroids, or cancer

Management in secondary care
- Possible investigations would be hysteroscopy, with polypectomy or endometrial biopsy as appropriate.
- Treat the cause by appropriate medicinal or surgical method.

Dysmenorrhoea

Dysmenorrhoea (painful periods) affects 40–70% of women of reproductive age, and affects daily activities in up to 10% of women.

Primary dysmenorrhoea is a cyclic pain associated with ovulatory cycles without demonstrable lesions affecting reproductive structures. The pain probably results from uterine contractions and ischaemia, mediated by prostaglandins produced in secretory endometrium. This disorder usually starts during adolescence and tends to decrease with age and after pregnancy.

Secondary, or acquired, dysmenorrhoea is pain with menses caused by demonstrable pathology. The commonest cause is endometriosis; adenomyosis may also cause it. Other causes include a tight cervical os secondary to surgery on the cervix. A pedunculated submucosal fibroid or an endometrial polyp extruding from the uterus can also cause cramping pain. PID may cause continuous low abdominal pain that increases with menses. Adhesions can also cause secondary dysmenorrhea. If present an IUCD occasionally can cause secondary dysmenorrhoea.

Diagnosis
When a patient presents with painful periods, it is important for the GP to distinguish between primary and secondary dysmenorrhoea. This can be achieved by appropriate history and examination.

Primary dysmenorrhoea is suggested by lower abdominal or pelvic pain that may radiate to the back and along the thighs occurring just prior to and/or during menstruation. Associated symptoms, such as headache, diarrhoea, nausea, and vomiting may be present and will usually date from about the time of menarche. There should be no abnormal findings on examination.

Secondary dysmenorrhoea, on the other hand, will often present with other gynaecological symptoms, such as dyspareunia, menorrhagia, and intermenstrual or post-coital bleeding. It usually has a later age of onset than primary dysmenorrhoea.

There may be abnormalities on examination, such as uterine tenderness or enlargement. However, the absence of abnormal findings does not necessarily exclude secondary dysmenorrhoea. The low abdominal pain present is usually crampy or colicky but can be a dull constant ache and radiate to the lower back or legs. The pain may start before or with menses and usually subsides after two days. Sometimes endometrial casts (membranous dysmenorrhoea) or clots are expelled. Other symptoms include headache, nausea (sometimes with vomiting), constipation or diarrhoea, and urinary symptoms.

Complications of dysmenorrhoea include psychological distress, absenteeism from school or work, and, if secondary dysmenorrhoea, complications from underlying pathology (e.g. infertility with endometriosis). It should be noted that irritable bowel syndrome is associated with dysmenorrhoea and may result in diagnostic confusion or inappropriate treatment.

Treatment
- With primary dysmenorrhoea, the woman should be reassured that her reproductive organs are normal. Many women will not need drugs once the condition is explained to them.
- Simple measures include use of a heating pad to the lower abdomen and back and use of TENS.
- Enquiry into use of over-the-counter medications is important, as many women with dysmenorrhoea self-medicate.
- Prostaglandin synthetase inhibitors, such as mefenamic acid (500mg tds orally during menses), and other NSAIDs (e.g. ibuprofen) are very effective.
- If contraception is also required then a combined oral contraceptive is ideal. Medroxyprogesterone acetate injection (Depo-Provera®) 150mg intramuscularly every 12 weeks can also be used to achieve the same purpose.
- IUCDs can cause dysmenorrhoea and may require removal if adequate pain relief is not provided with other treatments. The levonorgestrel-releasing intrauterine system coil appears to reduce dysmenorrhoea and may be an alternative if an IUCD is still desired.
- Anti-spasmodics, such as hyoscine butylbromide and alverine citrate, are licensed for the treatment of dysmenorrhoea, but there is a lack of evidence on their efficacy.
- Symptoms such as vomiting rarely require treatment with anti-emetics once the primary problem is treated.
- Alternative therapies are popular with many patients. There is some evidence that hypnosis is effective. Herbs and other phytomedicinal products are often tried by women for dysmenorrhoea. Evidence for their efficacy is very limited.

Indications for referral
- Secondary dysmenorrhoea suspected from history and/or examination.
- Women who fail to respond to standard drug treatments.
- Laparoscopy is indicated in cases of resistant dysmenorrhoea to diagnose disorders such as endometriosis.

- Presacral neurectomy or uterine nerve ablation is an option for women with resistant dysmenorrhoea, though evidence of efficacy is controversial.

Useful tips

○ It is important for the GP to differentiate between primary and secondary dysmenorrhoea, with the latter usually requiring specialist referral.
○ In primary dysmenorrhoea, explain the physiological basis for the symptoms and reassure the women that their reproductive organs are normal. Mefenamic acid will bring about symptomatic relief in 80% of women.

Amenorrhoea

Amenorrhoea is the absence of menstruation. This can be because either menses never began or later ceased. Primary amenorrhoea is usually diagnosed when menarche has not occurred by age 16. Secondary amenorrhoea is when menses has not occurred for six months or more in women who have had menses previously. The two conditions are considered separately below.

Primary amenorrhoea: causes and diagnosis

- Primary amenorrhoea often causes great anxiety, but in most patients puberty is later than expected, often as a familial trait. In these cases, reassurance is all that is needed.
- Other patients may have factors that cause primary amenorrhoea to arise prior to menarche.
- Imperforate hymen or other structural abnormalities of the genitalia are also causes.
- Structural or genetic causes are less common. It is important for the GP to assess if the patient has normal external secondary sexual characteristics. If there is abnormal development, examination and karyotyping may reveal Turner's syndrome or testicular feminisation.

Management in primary care

- Reassurance if the patient is late to enter puberty; e.g. because of familial reasons.
- In the case of genetic abnormalities such as Turner's syndrome or testicular feminisation, the aim is to help the patient to lead a normal life including functioning sexually, and, if possible, to enable her to reproduce if the woman desires.

Secondary amenorrhoea: causes

The incidence of secondary amenorrhoea (due to causes other than pregnancy) is about 4% in the general population. Amenorrhoea indicates failure of hypothalamic-pituitary-gonadal-uterine interaction to produce cyclic changes in the endometrium, resulting in menses.

There are many possible causes for missed or delayed menstruation:
- pregnancy
- lactation
- ovarian causes: premature menopause, radiotherapy or chemotherapy, androgen-producing tumours, and, rarely, polycystic ovaries
- stress or anxiety
- excessive prolonged exercise
- obesity or malnutrition and eating disorders like anorexia nervosa
- use of oral contraceptives (both combined and progestogen-only) as well as non-oral contraceptives such as Depo-Provera® and the levonorgestrel-releasing intrauterine system; 'post-pill amenorrhoea' is usually oligomenorrhoea masked by regular withdrawal bleeds
- severe systemic illness; e.g. renal failure
- hormonal imbalance
- thyroid disorders
- pituitary tumour
- uterine causes; e.g. Asherman's syndrome (uterine adhesions after a D+C of the uterus).

Diagnosis
Patients should be asked about abnormal growth and development or if there is any family history of genetic anomalies. Diet and exercise habits, lifestyle, and any environmental stresses or psychological symptoms should be asked about.

When taking a history it is important to assess if there are any other associated symptoms, such as headache, galactorrhea, visual loss, marked weight changes, dry vagina, hirsutism, voice changes, or breast size changes. A physical examination should be performed, including a pelvic examination. Physical and pelvic examinations must rule out pregnancy before other diagnostic testing begins.

The woman should be encouraged to discuss her anxieties and may be referred for psychological counselling if appropriate.

Diagnostic tests that may be performed
- Urinary pregnancy test.
- FSH and LH levels.
- Prolactin level.
- Thyroid function tests.

- Serum testosterone and DHEAS should be measured in hirsute women. High testosterone levels may suggest an androgen-producing tumour (e.g. of ovarian origin). High DHEAS levels may indicate an adrenal neoplasm.

Management in primary care
Changes in lifestyle should be suggested if stress, exercise, or weight loss or gain is perceived to be the problem. Referral for psychological assessment and counselling may be required if anxiety or stress is the cause.

Treatment depends on the cause of the amenorrhoea. If it is caused by another systemic disorder, normal menstrual function usually returns after the primary disorder is treated. For example, if the primary disorder is hyperthyroidism, then the amenorrhea will be cured when the thyroid disorder is treated.

If pregnancy is confirmed, arrange for routine antenatal care or termination of pregnancy as appropriate.

When to refer
It is not usually necessary to refer for a specialist opinion unless there has been at least six months' amenorrhoea. Referral should be seriously considered if no obvious cause is found by this stage.

Tests that may be required in secondary care
- Endometrial biopsy
- Karyotyping
- Skull X-ray and CT scan of the head if suspected pituitary tumour
- Progestational challenge to confirm the presence of normal endometrium

---

Useful points
○ Before any other investigations, always exclude pregnancy.
○ Consider referral to a specialist if amenorrhoea persists for more than six months and no obvious cause is found.

Premature Menopause (Premature Ovarian Failure)
Premature menopause is defined as ovarian failure in women below 40 years of age. Such women have high levels of circulating gonadotrophins (especially FSH) and low levels of oestradiol. It affects about 1% of women.

Premature menopause is most commonly due to surgical removal of the uterus and ovaries (surgical menopause). Other causes may be congenital (if the ovaries failed to develop) or familial (possibly due to an increased rate of disappearance of follicles), and chromosomal abnormalities (e.g. Turner's syndrome), the presence of ovarian antibodies, and damage to the ovaries (from infections such as the mumps or by radiotherapy or chemotherapy) should also be considered.

Diagnosis
A thorough history and examination should be undertaken. Often there is a family history of premature menopause and autoimmune conditions.

Investigations
The following investigations can be undertaken in primary care, but most are best undertaken by a specialist:
- gonadotrophin levels (high in all patients); oestradiol levels (low)
- karyotyping
- auto-antibody screen, such as anti-nuclear antibodies; anti-thyroid antibodies (and TSH to exclude thyroid problems); ESR and rheumatoid factor
- serum calcium and phosphorus to exclude hypoparathyroidism
- morning cortisol to rule out hypoadrenalism
- FBC, total protein, and albumin/globulin ratio.

Treatment
A common misperception is that premature menopause isn't a significant condition. In fact, for many sufferers, it can have a major impact in several ways. It may cause infertility, which can have a major effect not only for the woman but her family as well. Even for women who have already had children, this can represent a huge sense of loss, and many women can feel old before their time. If their doctor trivialises the problem, it can cause anxiety in some women. Apart from the likelihood of infertility, sufferers go through the same consequences of oestrogen deficiency as menopausal women over the age of 50, such as osteoporosis and heart disease. This oestrogen loss is even before these women have had the full benefits of oestrogen in their lives, such as maximal bone mass.

In the case of familial premature menopause, reassurance for the woman is important.

Women who have premature ovarian failure and do not want to become pregnant can be given HRT (see 'The Menopause and Hormone Replacement Therapy').

For those who desire pregnancy, an option is oocyte donation, with artificial cycles stimulated by exogenous oestrogen and progesterone, so that the oocytes fertilised in vitro can be transferred to an appropriately stimulated endometrium.

Further Reading

1. O'Brien PMS. Disorders of the menstrual cycle. In: Campbell S, Monga A (eds). *Gynaecology by Ten Teachers.* [17th ed.] London: Edward Arnold, 2000; pp 47–63.
2. O'Brien PMS. *Premenstrual Syndrome.* London: Blackwell Science, 1987.
3. Wyatt K. Premenstrual syndrome. *Clin Evid* 2002; **7:** 1739–1757.
4. Royal College of Obstetricians and Gynaecologists. *The Initial Management of Menorrhagia. Evidence-based Clinical Guidelines, No 1.* London: RCOG, 1998.
5. Duckitt K. Menorrhagia. *Clin Evid* 2002; **8:** 1934–1950.
6. Lethaby A, Augood C, Duckitt K. Nonsteroidal anti-inflammatory drugs for heavy menstrual bleeding (Cochrane Review). In: *The Cochrane Library,* Issue 2. Oxford: Update Software, 2002.
7. O'Brien S, Doyle M. Abnormal vaginal bleeding. In: Luesley DM (ed). *Common Conditions in Gynaecology: A Problem Solving Approach.* [1st ed.] London: Chapman and Hall, 1997; pp 57–80.
8. Wilson M, Farquhar C. Dysmenorrhoea. *Clin Evid* 2002; **7:** 1639–1653.
9. McIver B, Romanski SA, Nippoldt TB. Evaluation and management of amenorrhea. *Mayo Clin Proc* 1997; **72(12):** 1161–1169.

Useful Websites

- Recommendations arising from the Study Group on Disorders of the Menstrual Cycle, RCOG. URL: http://www.rcog.org.uk/mainpages.asp?PageID=442.
- The Initial Management of Menorrhagia, Royal College of Obstetricians and Gynaecologists. URL:http://www.rcog.org.uk/guidelines.asp?PageID=108&GuidelineID=28.
- Women's Health. URL: http://www.womenshealthlondon.org.uk/.
- National Association for Premenstrual Syndrome. URL: http://www.pms.org.uk/.
- The Premature Ovarian Failure Support Group. URL: http://www.pofsupport.org/.

The Menopause and Hormone Replacement Therapy

Dr Manish Latthe

Introduction

The menopause is the permanent cessation of the menstrual cycle in women. It is the ending of a phase of gradual decline in ovarian function that marks the end of the reproductive years. Although the menopause occurs in all women, each woman's experience of it is different. With increasing life expectancy, diagnosing and managing the menopause will continue to be a major part of a GP's workload.

Menopause may be natural, artificial, or premature. A natural menopause is deemed to have occurred after 12 months of cessation of menstruation in a woman aged 45 years or older. The average age of occurrence in the UK is 51 years. Smoking has been shown to lower the age of menopause.

Artificial, or surgical, menopause occurs when the ovaries are removed. Between 10–20% of women who have had a hysterectomy with ovaries conserved have early menopause, typically between one to four years earlier than a natural menopause.

Premature menopause is discussed in 'Abnormalities of Menstruation'.

Physiology and Endocrinology

Hormonal changes

As a woman approaches the menopause, her ovaries' response to pituitary gonadotrophins (LH and FSH) decreases. This at first causes shorter follicular phases (i.e. shorter menstrual cycles) with fewer ovulations, decreased progesterone production, and less cycle regularity. Then the follicle fails to respond and does not produce oestrogen. Without oestrogen feedback, LH and FSH levels rise substantially, while circulating levels of oestrogens and progesterone fall. This transitional phase is called the climacteric or perimenopause. In postmenopausal women, androgens are converted to oestrogens in the periphery (e.g. in fat cells), thereby accounting for most of the circulating oestrogen.

Diagnosis

About 75% of women will not experience any troubling symptoms when they reach the menopause. Nevertheless, in most cases it is possible to diagnose if a woman is peri- or postmenopausal by taking a detailed history.

Menstrual irregularities are common before periods finally stop, often because cycles are anovulatory. Initially, there may be more frequent periods or heavier periods than usual before they finally cease.

In the early stages of oestrogen depletion, most symptoms are either neuroendocrine or urogenital:

Neuroendocrine symptoms	Urogenital symptoms
hot flushes	urinary incontinence
night sweats	dyspareunia
palpitations	vaginal dryness
depression	prolapse
emotional changes	urinary infections
irritability	
headaches	
lethargy	

Other changes include forgetfulness, reduced libido, thinning of the skin, hair changes, sleeping difficulties, musculoskeletal symptoms (e.g. joint pains), and reduced mastalgia symptoms.

Investigations are not required in most cases. However, if the diagnosis is not clear from the history, hormone levels can be checked. As mentioned, FSH and LH levels rise while oestrogen levels fall, though they can fluctuate for up to 12 months after the menopause. However, hormone levels are not always diagnostic and levels can change from one day to another. They may help to gauge the onset of menopause when a woman has had a hysterectomy or if menopause is suspected in women under the age of 40.

Management of the perimenopause

In every woman who presents with symptoms at this time, there are three main factors to be discussed:
1. An explanation of the changes that occur during the menopause.
2. General health education about healthy diet and lifestyle.
3. The benefits and risks of HRT.

Clinical Consequences of Oestrogen Depletion and the Benefits of Hormone Replacement Therapy

Bone loss

An significant effect of oestrogen depletion is the increase in rate of bone loss in women, particularly in the early stages of the menopause. The current evidence suggests that while on HRT, bone mineral density is maintained in the spine, proximal femur, and radius. The WHI study has established that the risk of hip fracture is reduced in women on HRT, with a relative risk of 0.66.

Cardiovascular risk

Previously, many doctors advised patients that HRT lowered the risk of an adverse cardiovascular event, but this advice was based on flawed studies (so-called healthy cohort effect). Recent studies have shown no benefit. HERS, which is the largest study of the role of secondary prevention of HRT in women who have suffered with coronary heart disease, found no preventive cardiovascular benefit. In fact, the risk of a cardiovascular event in this group rose in the first year and then subsequently fell. HERS II was a follow-up study to evaluate the effects of longer-duration hormone therapy. The trend towards a reduced risk of heart attacks did not persist with additional follow-up. Over almost seven years, combining HERS and HERS II, there was no reduction in risk among women taking hormones.

Senile dementia and memory loss

In one meta-analysis, HRT was associated with a 34% reduction in the risk of dementia (LeBlanc et al, 2001). Subsequent epidemiological studies are inconsistent. HRT may be associated with a reduced risk of dementia, but it has no effect on the established disease.

Colon cancer

Recently, HRT has been postulated as reducing the risk of colon cancer. The best evidence to date is from the WHI study, which states an absolute benefit of five cancers prevented per 10,000 women per year. A meta-analysis of 25 trials found that there was a 33% reduction in colon cancer risk.

Hormone Replacement Therapy and Risks Associated with its Use

The benefits of HRT are noted above. However, HRT is not suitable for all women; those without symptoms may have little to gain. When prescribing HRT it is important to remember that each woman has a unique risk profile that might lead to varying benefit from HRT. An inflexible policy applied to all women will not be effective.

Aims of therapy

When prescribing HRT we should aim to reduce the symptoms and prevent the disorders arising from oestrogen depletion, while trying to avoid causing disorders that may be common with oestrogen therapy, such as endometrial and breast cancer.

Symptoms associated with hormone replacement therapy
Oestrogen side-effects
Minor symptoms such as breast tenderness, leg cramps at night, nausea, and mild fluid retention are the most common oestrogen side-effects. These can be improved by reducing the oestrogen dose or by using an alternative route of administration. There is no scientific evidence to support the belief that there is any weight gain due to HRT (either unopposed oestrogen or combined therapy) above that which normally is gained during the menopause.

Progestogen side-effects
Progestogen side-effects include premenstrual syndrome-type symptoms, such as mood swings, irritability, and depression, as well as breast tenderness, fluid retention, and abdominal bloating. Changing the type of progestogen can help these symptoms. The intake of progestogens can be reduced by prescribing it at a lower dose or for the least number of days (i.e. 10–12 days). It is possible that the less androgenic dydrogesterone and medroxyprogesterone acetate cause fewer side-effects, such as acne, than levonorgestrel or norethisterone.

Bleeding
Withdrawal of cyclical progestogen in combined HRT will cause a withdrawal bleed that may be heavy or painful in some women. This is a major cause of poor compliance. Many women prefer to use 'period-free' HRT preparations (see p25). If irregular bleeding persists for more than three months it should be investigated to exclude underlying pathology. Investigations in secondary care may include pelvic ultrasonography, endometrial biopsy, and hysteroscopy to diagnose underlying endometrial pathology such as polyps, hyperplasia, or carcinoma.

Disorders associated with hormone replacement therapy
Breast cancer
Previously, it was thought that the cumulative excess of breast cancers were two per 1000 during the first five years of HRT, six per 1000 for HRT use for ten years, and 12 per 1000 for HRT use over 15 years. However, at the time of publication, new research published in the *Lancet* has shown the risk to be considerably higher. The Million Women Study is an observational study of UK women, aged 50–64 years, which was designed to investigate the risk of breast cancer while using the different types of HRT. The data showed that in women aged 50–64 there are about 20 breast cancer cases diagnosed per 1000 women, and for the same number of women using oestrogen-only HRT for ten years there will be an additional five cases; combined HRT adds another 19 cases. Also, the research showed that users of HRT had a 22% higher risk of dying from breast cancer compared with women who had never taken it. The risk of breast cancer increased with longer use of HRT, but the effect seemed to wear off within a few years of stopping treatment. The researchers estimated that use of HRT in women aged 50–64 years has resulted in 20,000

extra cases of breast cancer over the past decade, of which 15,000 would be associated with combined HRT.

Endometrial cancer

Unopposed oestrogen therapy can cause proliferation of the endometrium, which may develop to carcinoma. The risk is significantly reduced by the addition of a progestogen to the regimen. It appears that at least ten days progestogen exposure per cycle is required to reduce the risk of oestrogen-associated endometrial cancer.

Venous thromboembolism

The excess risk of developing deep vein thrombosis is estimated to be between 1-2-in-10,000 per year (i.e. from 1 case per 10,000 women per year in non-users to between 2 and 3 per 10,000 women per year in users). Risk is greatest in the first year of taking HRT, declining thereafter.

Cerebrovascular accidents

Initially, studies had found no consistent evidence; however, the WHI study has suggested increased risk of strokes in women on HRT, with a relative risk of 1.41.

Epithelial ovarian cancer

The incidence of ovarian cancer is greater in well-educated women and those in higher socio-economic groups, who are most likely to use HRT. No studies have found that using oestrogen for less than ten years is associated with an increased risk. Overall, the results of the epidemiological studies do not currently suggest that the risk of epithelial ovarian cancer is increased by the use of HRT.

Summary of risks and benefits

The WHI study focused on defining the risks and benefits of strategies that could potentially reduce the incidence of heart disease, breast and colorectal cancer, and fractures in post-menopausal women. The HRT preparation used was combined oestrogen and progestogen in one daily tablet containing conjugated equine oestrogen 0.625mg, and medroxyprogesterone acetate 2.5mg. The data shows the relative and absolute risk of combined HRT vs. placebo group (*n* = 16,608) over 5.2 years (Grady *et al*, 2002).

Practical Prescribing of Hormone Replacement Therapy

Types of hormone replacement therapy

The hormones used in HRT are oestrogen and progestogen. Prolonged use of unopposed oestrogen can cause endometrial hyperplasia and carcinoma (see above). Thus, women with a uterus should be given oestrogen with some form of progestogen to protect the endometrium. On the other hand, women who have had a hysterectomy can be prescribed oestrogen alone.

Event	Relative risk	Increased absolute risk per 10,000 women/year	Increased absolute benefit per 10,000 women/year
MI	1.29	7	–
CVA	1.41	8	–
Breast cancer	1.26	8	–
Colorectal cancer	0.63	–	6
Hip fractures	0.66	–	5

- The risks were coronary heart disease (increased from 30 to 37 cases per 10,000 women per year), stroke (increased from 21 to 29 cases per 10,000 women per year), and breast cancer (increased from 30 to 38 cases per 10,000 women per year).
- The benefits were a reduction in colorectal cancer (reduced from 16 to 10 cases per 10,000 women per year) and hip fracture (reduced from 15 to 10 cases per 10,000 women per year).

Source: *JAMA* 2002; **288(3):** 321–333. Copyright© 2002, American Medical Association. All rights reserved.

Oestrogens

Oestrogen can be either natural (oestradiol, oestrone, oestriol) or synthetic (ethinyloestradiol, mestranol). The former make up the majority of HRT preparations; in particular, conjugated equine oestrogens (they are extracted from the urine of pregnant mares and contain about 60% oestrone) are the market leaders in oral oestrogen preparations in the UK. Some women may prefer not to use HRT preparations containing these oestrogens. The synthetic oestrogens have been associated with an increased risk of venous thrombosis.

Routes of administration for oestrogen

1. Oral oestrogens are the most popular route for HRT users in the UK. They are generally convenient and inexpensive and can be easily altered if necessary. A correspondingly higher dose of oral oestrogen is needed to achieve the same effect as a lower dose given via a non-oral route because of the first-pass effect through the liver. Oral oestrogens can cause mild gastrointestinal side-effects.
2. Transdermal oestrogens, i.e. patches or gels, are convenient and popular. The matrix patches are well tolerated. Transdermal oestrogens avoid the first-pass effect in the liver and are generally a preferable route in women with hepato-biliary and other gastrointestinal diseases. Natural oestradiol can be given via this route and in a lower dose than oral preparations. They are more expensive than oral preparations. Usually given twice weekly, there are now once-weekly preparations as well. Occasionally, they can cause local skin reactions.
3. Subcutaneous oestrogen implants are less popular. They can be given at the time of hysterectomy and oophorectomy. They release hormone (oestradiol) slowly over several months; 25, 50, and 100mg pellets are available but 100mg should not be

used routinely. A testosterone implant may be inserted simultaneously (improves libido). Insertion is performed under local anaesthetic, usually into the anterior abdominal wall or buttock, and repeated every six months or so when symptoms have returned. Tachyphylaxis – i.e. the effect that each time an implant is fitted, the symptoms return more quickly despite supraphysiological hormone levels – is a major problem only with this type of oestrogen delivery. In these cases, women have to be 'weaned off' implants and onto another type of oestrogen therapy.

4. Vaginal oestrogens are used to provide low-dose therapy to improve urogenital symptoms with minimal systemic absorption. Most low-dose vaginal oestrogens are recommended for only three to six months' continuous use; if used for longer, they should be combined with cyclical progestogens to reduce the (small) risk of endometrial hyperplasia. They are useful for women who have contraindications to systemic HRT. Also available is an oestrogen intravaginal ring that delivers systemic oestradiol for three months, suitable for women that have had a hysterectomy. The product maintains very stable levels of oestrogen, and is useful for urogenital symptoms in particular.

5. Nasal spray. Recently, a nasal spray providing oestradiol has been marketed. This preparation appears to be as effective as the other oestrogen delivery routes and in time may become a popular route of administering HRT. It is marketed as being useful for prompt symptomatic relief of hot flushes and night sweats. It is, however, more expensive than oral oestrogen.

Progestogens
For those women who still have their uterus, progestogen must be added to prevent endometrial carcinoma, usually for at least 10–12 days per cycle.

Routes of administration for progestogens
1. Oral. Various synthetically manufactured progestogens are used (norethisterone, norgestrel, dydrogesterone, medroxyprogesterone acetate) for 12–14 days per cycle. Usually, the HRT is provided in packs containing oestrogen pills for the first half of the cycle and pills containing both oestrogen and progestogen for the second half of the cycle.

2. Transdermal patches. Combined oestrogen and progestogen transdermal patches are available; the matrix type patches are considered superior to the reservoir type patches, as they adhere better and are better tolerated.

3. Progestogen-releasing intrauterine systems can be delivered via a hormone-releasing intrauterine system with systemic oestrogen. At the time of writing, the levonorgestrel-releasing intrauterine system is not yet licensed in the UK for use as part of HRT regimens but is licensed in other countries for this use. A smaller intrauterine system suitable for use in postmenopausal women is in phase II clinical trials and is expected to be licensed as the progesterone arm of HRT in the UK in the near future.

Three-monthly bleed hormone replacement therapy
Progestogens can be given for either 12–14 days each month giving a monthly bleed (as explained above) or for 14 days every three months giving a three-monthly bleed, which some women prefer. There is some concern about the protection of the endometrium with this regimen and hence it is recommended to be used for two to three years during transition towards menopause.

Period-free hormone replacement therapy
Another option for postmenopausal women is the period-free HRT regimens or continuous combined therapy, where oestrogen and progestogen are taken together every day. These continuous combined HRT preparations are suitable for women who are at least one year past their last menstrual period or over the age of 54. Use of period-free HRT improves compliance, but a common side-effect in the first few months of use is irregular spotting. If this persists for longer than six months, referral to a specialist for further investigation is required. Unlike the sequential preparations, which have a double charge, these preparations only incur a single prescription charge.

Contraindications
Absolute contraindications
- Past or present (or suspected) oestrogen-dependent neoplasia
- Severe liver disease
- Undiagnosed vaginal bleeding
- Pregnancy

Relative contraindications
- *Breast cancer.* Oestrogens are causally related to breast cancer. Most breast specialists advise against use of HRT because of the possible increased risk of recurrence, however trials have failed to demonstrate an increase in either the rate of tumour recurrence or the rate of death (we do not yet have the results of RCTs, which will provide better evidence regarding the safety of HRT in women that have had breast cancer). Until we know more, women who have been recently diagnosed with breast cancer are advised not to take HRT. In women with a strong family history of breast cancer (and therefore at a higher risk themselves) many would advise that HRT use should be limited to five years at most.
- *Ovarian cancer.* The evidence suggests that there is no increased risk of ovarian cancer associated with HRT, and no reason for women not to restart HRT after the cancer has been treated.
- *Endometrial cancer.* The risk of endometrial cancer is increased in women using HRT. Results from observational studies suggest that after treatment of endometrial cancer, women who take oestrogen do better than those who do not, and those with early-stage disease or who have had no recurrence for five years could be prescribed HRT and no longer require progestogens because they have undergone hysterectomy.

- *Diabetes.* There is no evidence that HRT is associated with increased morbidity or mortality in diabetic women, but different types of oestrogen and progestogen appear to have different effects on carbohydrate metabolism (e.g. 1.25mg/day conjugated equine oestrogens can cause a significant deterioration in insulin resistance). Dydrogesterone with oestradiol is sometimes recommended as a first choice for these women.
- *Family history of VTE.* If it were associated with oestrogen use (e.g. COCP) or with a precipitating factor such as obesity that is still present, it would be best to avoid HRT. A thrombophilia screen may be useful in other cases. If there is no obvious cause, and the woman is fully counselled of the increased risks, then she may be prescribed HRT, avoiding the oral route to shun the first-pass effect and starting with the lowest possible dose of oestrogen. Some haematologists advise using warfarin or low-dose aspirin for women with a positive thrombophilia screen who want to take oestrogen.
- *Hypertension and ischaemic heart disease.* HRT is not usually associated with a negative effect on the blood pressure either in women being treated for hypertension or in normotensive women, though very occasionally it can increase blood pressure. The transdermal route using the lowest possible dose to achieve symptom relief would be safest. Following the HERS and WHI reports it is now advised that HRT should not be initiated solely for the prevention of coronary heart disease.
- *Depression.* Oestrogen and androgen have a generally positive effect on mood, while progestogens have a negative effect. In a perimenopausal woman complaining of low mood, a trial of HRT can be undertaken, but if this is not effective in alleviating low mood, then antidepressant therapy or referral to psychiatric services should be considered. In women with clinically diagnosed depression who are on antidepressants, HRT may be of added benefit and is not contraindicated.
- *Endometriosis.* The oestrogen in HRT may stimulate recurrence of endometriosis occasionally and this should be made clear to women suffering with this condition. Patients who have undergone hysterectomy and bilateral salpingoophorectomy for this condition do not have any contraindications for oestrogen replacement. If there is risk of residual disease after hysterectomy, a combined preparation is advisable.
- *Migraine.* Some women find that HRT causes an increase in the frequency and severity of migraines, while others find the opposite. It is worth a trial of HRT to see what effect it has.

Prescribing hormone replacement therapy
Counselling patients

This is the most important aspect of prescribing HRT. The woman needs to be counselled fully regarding the benefits and risks of HRT, and made aware of the different types of preparations available, as well as the alternatives to HRT (see p29). She should be given the opportunity to make an informed decision. Also, contraception needs to be discussed (if appropriate).

When to start hormone replacement therapy
In women with menopausal symptoms who are still menstruating, HRT can be started within a few days of the beginning of the next menstrual period. In those who have finished menstruating, it can be started at any time.

HRT can be started at a later age as well; for example, women above the age of 60. Some would argue that this is more beneficial in preventing osteoporosis, as they may be less active then.

Most GPs would prescribe the cheaper oral preparations first, depending on the products that they are used to prescribing and the presence of any local guidelines or protocols for prescribing HRT.

Investigations before starting
- Hormone levels. A high FSH level (>30) will confirm the diagnosis of menopause where there is a doubt clinically.
- Cervical screening and mammography should be undertaken as per the national screening programmes.
- Thrombophilia screen only if indicated by history.
- Thyroid function tests only if indicated.
- Lipid levels only if indicated.
- Endometrial sampling and pelvic ultrasonography should be performed if the GP is concerned about symptoms suggesting endometrial abnormalities (e.g. menorrhagia, intermenstrual bleeding).
- Bone density screening is only for those considered to be at high risk of osteoporosis; not for routine screening.

Examination
- Blood pressure is routinely performed.
- Breast self-examination should be encouraged and taught if necessary.
- Pelvic examination is not usually required.

Monitoring hormone replacement therapy
Most GPs will prescribe a three-month course of HRT, and if the woman remains well will follow with six-monthly prescriptions. At follow-up consultations, most GPs will assess the following:
- any side-effects from HRT
- blood pressure
- mammography and cervical smears are being done
- weight to assess any gain
- breast examination if the woman has any concerns; self-examinations should be encouraged if possible.

Contraception
Hormone replacement therapy will not provide contraception and the recommended advice is to provide contraception to women on HRT for two years if they have started treatment under the age of 50, or for one year if above the age of 50. Since fertility is relatively low in perimenopausal women, doctors usually recommend barrier methods, IUCD, or the progestogen-only pill as suitable forms of contraception.

When to stop hormone replacement therapy
There remain differing views about how long to continue HRT. Assuming that there are no side-effects, most GPs will prescribe HRT for between five to ten years after the normal age of menopause (average age of occurrence in the UK is 51 years). If used for longer, the risks are thought to outweigh the benefits. The duration will be longer in women who have had a premature or surgical menopause, but these women can be reassured that the risk of breast cancer with HRT is based only on women over 50 years. It should be remembered that many women stop HRT without medical advice.

Alternatives to Hormone Replacement Therapy
Selective oestrogen receptor modulators
This is a newer class of drugs now in use in the management of menopause. The first such drug is raloxifene and it combines both oestrogenic and anti-oestrogenic activity; it has differing effects on oestrogen receptors in various tissues. It is an oestrogen agonist to bone and is licensed for the prevention of osteoporotic fractures. However, it is anti-oestrogenic in breast and endometrial tissue and so reduces the risk of breast cancer and endometrial proliferation. On the negative side, women taking raloxifene may suffer increased vasomotor symptoms. It is most suitable for older postmenopausal women and those at increased risk of breast cancer.

Clonidine
Clonidine is a drug licensed for treatment of menopausal flushing. It is an alpha-blocker and is also used in the treatment of hypertension. It has no effect on osteoporosis.

Tibolone
Tibolone is a synthetic oral steroid with oestrogenic, progestogenic, and androgenic actions. It is licensed as an alternative to conventional continuous combined HRT. It is indicated for osteoporosis prophylaxis, and it can control the vasomotor, urogenital, and psychological symptoms in menopause, but there is little evidence to show that it prevents coronary heart disease. Adverse effects reported include abnormal vaginal bleeding and headache, besides other less common ones.

Bisphosphonates
Bisphosphonates are a well-established family of non-hormonal drugs used to prevent and treat postmenopausal osteoporosis. They are adsorbed onto hydroxyapatite crystals in

bone, slowing both their rate of growth and dissolution, and so reducing the rate of bone turnover. Bisphosphonates are poorly absorbed and must be taken on an empty stomach. As well as medication, it should be remembered that adequate calcium, vitamin D, and exercise are also important for maintaining bone health.

Herbal medicines and phyto-oestrogens

With more women concerned about the risks associated with conventional HRT, there has been a great increase in interest in alternative therapies, such as herbal medicines. A large range of herbal preparations have been promoted for the treatment of menopausal symptoms; for many of them there is no scientific evidence to prove they are effective. Herbs promoted for treatment of menopause include black cohosh, chaste tree, St John's Wort, evening primrose oil, dong quai, wild yam cream, ginseng, kava kava, and red clover.

However, the most effective compounds are considered to be phyto-oestrogens. These are non-steroidal plant-derived compounds that have a mild oestrogenic activity. Soy products are the commonest source. There is a lack of conclusive evidence of their effectiveness, but several RCTs produced results that showed that soy reduced some oestrogen deficiency symptoms, particularly hot-flushes, compared with placebo or other controls.

Overall, phyto-oestrogens do seem to have some benefits for postmenopausal women. There seem to be relatively few risks with phyto-oestrogens, unless taken in very high doses, when they will carry the risks associated with oestrogen treatment itself. There is also some evidence that they may suppress endogenous oestrogen production.

Use of herbal medicines requires much more scientific evidence before they can be recommended.

Osteoporosis: Prevention and Treatment

Osteoporosis was defined by WHO in 1994 as a 'progressive systemic skeletal disease characterised by low bone mass and microarchitectural deterioration of bone tissue, with a consequent increase in bone fragility and susceptibility to fracture'. It is a major clinical problem in the UK. Fractures of the wrist, the spine, and especially the hip cause significant morbidity and mortality. At particular risk are women with early menopause, a family history of osteoporosis, thin habitus, a previous fragility fracture, those on long-term corticosteroids, and smokers.

The main diagnostic technique is DEXA at the hip for diagnosis and at the spine for assessing response to treatment.

Prevention
- Lifestyle factors include weight-bearing exercise, adequate intake of calcium in the diet, and stopping smoking; preventing falls is also important. Reducing alcohol intake may help.
- HRT is very effective in the prevention of osteoporosis in postmenopausal women while they are taking it.
- Alternatives are bisphosphonates (e.g. etidronate with calcium) and selective oestrogen receptor modulators (raloxifene). Calcium and vitamin D supplements are useful in the elderly but are generally less effective.

Treatment
All treatments are effective only while being taken, with no residual benefit once stopped.
- HRT
- Bisphosphonates
- Calcium (with or without vitamin D)
- Calcitonin
- Vitamin D metabolites: calcitriol and alphacalcidol

Well Woman Clinics
Well woman clinics are often the setting in which patients receive counselling and treatment for the menopause. These clinics are a well-established part of medical practice in the UK. They have been set up in a variety of settings, including in primary care, in hospitals, and sometimes as stand-alone clinics. In the primary care setting, they are run by practice nurses and/or GPs. They can have a wide variety of roles, depending on the setting and the target population, but a common feature is that they usually offer a longer consultation time than the woman would normally get with her GP and more in the way of screening and counselling is offered.

Many well woman clinics offer screening to enable the early detection and treatment of breast and cervical cancer; i.e. a breast examination and cervical smear could be offered. Counselling and monitoring of HRT is another role. The latter could involve breast examination, checking blood pressure, and asking about contraception if appropriate.

Well woman clinics are a good opportunity to ask about a woman's current state of health, family history, smoking habits, alcohol consumption, diet, exercise levels, and contraception.

Other tasks that are often performed include:
- height and weight measurements
- blood pressure
- breast examination and instruction on breast self-examination

- cervical smear
- pelvic examination
- blood tests such as FBC to assess if anaemic, rubella status
- urinalysis.

Useful tips

○ Before prescribing HRT it is extremely important to ensure that the woman is fully aware of the known benefits and risks associated with treatment. It is usually better to give the information and allow the woman to decide. Treatment needs to be tailored to each individual.

○ Prescribing HRT should be for clear clinical reasons; e.g. treatment of menopausal symptoms. HRT will not be suitable for all women and other options should be offered if appropriate.

○ HRT increases the relative risk of myocardial infarction, cerebrovascular accidents, and breast cancer.

○ Hormone levels during the perimenopause period are highly variable and therefore rarely of use for diagnostic purposes. In most cases the diagnosis is usually clear from the history.

○ Non-hysterectomised women must have progestogen in addition to oestrogen for at least 10–12 days per cycle.

○ Phyto-oestrogens have been shown to be useful in the treatment of menopause symptoms, but little evidence exists for the herbal medications currently widely used as alternatives to conventional HRT.

Further Reading

1. Rymer J, Morris EP. Extracts from "Clinical Evidence": Menopausal symptoms. *BMJ* 2000; **321**: 1516–1519.
2. MacLennan A, Lester S, Moore V. Oral estrogen replacement therapy versus placebo for hot flushes: a systematic review. *Climacteric* 2001; **4(1)**: 58–74.
3. Burkman RT, Collins JA, Greene RA. Current perspectives on benefits and risks of hormone replacement therapy. *Am J Obstet Gynecol* 2001; **185(2 Suppl)**: S13–23.
4. Grady D, Herrington D, Bittner V, *et al.* Cardiovascular disease outcomes during 6.8 years of hormone therapy: Heart and Estrogen/progestin Replacement Study follow-up (HERS II). *JAMA* 2002; **288(1)**: 49–57.
5. Writing Group for the Women's Health Initiative Investigators. Risks and benefits of estrogen plus progestin in healthy postmenopausal women: principal results from the Women's Health Initiative randomized controlled trial. *JAMA* 2002; **288(3)**: 321–333.
6. LeBlanc ES, Janowsky J, Chan BK, Nelson HD. Hormone replacement therapy and cognition: systematic review and meta-analysis. *JAMA* 2001; **285(11)**: 1489–1499.
7. Wells M, Sturdee DW, Barlow DH, *et al.* Effect on endometrium of long term

continuous combined oestrogen-progestogen replacement therapy: follow up study. *BMJ* 2002; **325:** 239.

8. Royal College of Obstetricians and Gynaecologists. *Hormone replacement therapy/ venous thromboembolism.* [Clinical Green Top Guidelines, No 19.] London: RCOG, 1998.

9. Lethaby A, Farquhar C, Sarkis A, *et al.* Hormone replacement therapy in postmenopausal women: endometrial hyperplasia and irregular bleeding (Cochrane Review). In: *The Cochrane Library,* Issue 1. Oxford: Update Software, 2002.

10. Davis SR. Phytoestrogen therapy for menopausal symptoms? *BMJ* 2001; **323:** 354–355.

11. Royal College of Physicians, Bone and Tooth Society of Great Britain. *Clinical guidelines for prevention and treatment. Update on pharmacological interventions and an algorithm for management.* London: Royal College of Physicians, 2000.

12. National Osteoporosis Society. *Guidance on the prevention and management of corticosteroid induced osteoporosis.* Bath: NOS, 1998.

13. Million Women Study Collaborators. Breast cancer and hormone replacement therapy in the Million Women Study. *Lancet* 2003; **362:** 419–427.

Useful Websites

- Summary and Recommendations of the Report "Osteoporosis – Clinical Guidelines for the Prevention and Treatment" (Royal College of Physicians).
  URL: http://www.doh.gov.uk/osteorep.htm.
- Educational resource site for professionals and patients (US-based) – Obgyn.net.
  URL: http://www.obgyn.net/meno/meno.asp.
- British Menopause Society. URL: http://www.the-bms.org/.
- The National Osteoporosis Society (NOS). URL: http://www.nos.org.uk/.
- Women's Health provides health information on gynaecological health issues including HRT and menopause. URL: http://www.womenshealthlondon.org.uk/.
- Women's Health Concern, PO Box 2126, Marlow, Bucks SL7 2RY. Helpline: 01628 483 612.

Incontinence and Prolapse

Mr Philip Tooz Hobson and Dr Samantha Pretlove

Introduction

Incontinence is a common problem, which although rarely life threatening can be profoundly disabling with a significant impact on day-to-day activity, social interactions, perceptions of well-being, and reduction in quality of life. Incontinence has been viewed in the past as a natural part of ageing or a consequence of having children and a condition that most women just have to put up with. A shift in women's expectations that they should be able to remain continent plus less embarrassment mean that increasing numbers of women now present to their GP with incontinence. New surgical techniques and drugs offer women effective treatment for their incontinence and help with tips on improving their quality of life and dealing with any problems that remain.

ICS definition of urinary incontinence:
Involuntary loss of urine that is a social or hygienic problem.

Prevalence varies widely in the literature and probably depends on which populations are included in the studies – e.g. hospital inpatients or nursing home residents – and the methods used to collect the data – e.g. interview or postal questionnaire – as embarrassment still plays a part. Estimates suggest 20-30% of the female population experience involuntary leakage of urine, but only 7-12% regard it as a problem and between 1–4% find that it restricts their daily activities. A recent (unpublished) MRC study suggests that in the UK, the average GP will have 50 patients with clinically significant and disabling incontinence.

Traditionally, assessment and treatment of prolapse, rather than incontinence, has been one of the mainstays of gynaecology. It is now becoming recognised that in many cases the patient's incontinence is far harder to treat than any concomitant prolapse and the emphasis should be reversed. Therefore, women presenting with prolapse should have underlying urinary problems excluded, after which treatment should then be focused on any incontinence. It is with this in mind that in this chapter, incontinence is discussed before and in far greater detail than pelvic organ prolapse.

The ICS has recently changed the terminology used to describe incontinence. The new terminology will be used throughout this chapter.

Previous terminology	ICS recommended terminology
Stress incontinence	Stress urinary incontinence
Urge incontinence	Urge urinary incontinence or sensory urgency
Detrusor instability	Idiopathic detrusor overactivity
Detrusor hyperreflexia	Neurogenic detrusor overactivity
Genuine stress incontinence	Urodynamic stress incontinence

The Bladder

The bladder is a hollow muscular organ that acts as a compliant reservoir. It is situated behind the pubic symphysis. The detrusor is made of smooth muscle fibres running in all directions. When the bladder contracts it reduces its diameter simultaneously in all directions.

The Urethra

The urethra is a hollow tube, 3-5cm long, that connects the bladder to the outside world. It is located under the pubic symphysis and travels through the pelvic diaphragm anterior to the vagina. It is lined with epithelium under which runs a rich vascular plexus that contributes to the urethral pressure. A layer of circular muscle surrounds the vascular plexus. This is coterminous with the detrusor muscle but separate to it.

The muscle in the urethra (sometimes termed the intrinsic sphincter mechanism) and the levator ani (the extrinsic sphincter mechanism) must combine to exert a pressure greater than that in the bladder to maintain continence. The proximal urethra is also supported by the pubourethral ligaments that attach it to the pubic symphysis.

Innervation of the Lower Urinary Tract

The detrusor is innervated by S2-S4 parasympathetic efferent fibres via the hypogastic plexus. There are also β-adrenergic receptors in bladder dome and neck and α-adrenergic receptors in bladder neck and urethra. The sympathetic outflow T10-L2 either acts directly on β receptors or inhibits parasympathetic excitatory supply to make the detrusor contract. Visceral afferent fibres that travel with the thoracolumbar and sacral efferents give the sensation of fullness with bladder distension.

Taking History

In order to obtain an accurate history it is important that the woman feels supported and that her symptoms are not dismissed. A comprehensive urogynaecological history can be divided into symptoms, risk factors, and quality of life issues. A full medical history and drug history are also important, as co-morbidity may influence symptoms.

It is very important that the possibility of a bladder tumour is excluded. Macroscopic haematuria or a history of a tumour should prompt early referral.

Symptoms
- Urgency
- Dysuria
- Frequency
- Nocturia
- Stress

ICS definition of urge urinary incontinence:
The complaint of involuntary leakage accompanied by, or immediately preceded by, urgency.

A good understanding of the significance of the patient's symptoms allows more precise and focused management. With **mixed** stress and urge symptoms, finding out which came first can be helpful. For example, a woman with stress incontinence alone initially may start emptying her bladder more frequently to reduce the amount of leakage when she coughs or sneezes. Her bladder gradually becomes accustomed to only containing small amounts of urine and she develops urgency when she tries to fill her bladder. Asking questions such as 'Can you watch a whole episode of EastEnders/Coronation Street without going to pass water?' can sometimes better elucidate the severity of frequency. **Bed-wetting** as a child is suggestive of detrusor overactivity. In women complaining of **nocturia** it is important to establish why they wake up, as sometimes depression or insomnia present as nocturia.

Risk factors for urinary incontinence
- *Female sex.* Risk increased two to three times when compared with men.
- *Age.* Although incontinence can occur at any age, it becomes much more common over the age of 70 and the severity of the incontinence also increases.
- *Pregnancy and childbirth.* Pregnancy, vaginal birth, forceps delivery, a prolonged active second stage, and large babies all increase the frequency of urinary incontinence, both immediately postpartum and later in life. Caesarean section does not necessarily prevent incontinence.
- *Menopause.* The reduction in oestrogen reduces the vascularity in the urethra and the surrounding connective tissue as well as the vulva and vagina. This can cause weakness in the fascia and ligaments, leading to urinary incontinence and pelvic organ prolapse.
- *Smoking.* Raises the risk of incontinence two to three times and also increases coughing, precipitating incontinence.
- *Obesity.*

Quality of life

Quality of life questionnaires are a useful adjunct to more traditional history taking. They are easy to complete and show how areas such as domestic tasks, work, exercise, social life, travelling, sleep, and intercourse are affected by incontinence. Having a formal questionnaire with every patient complaining of incontinence in primary care may not always be realistic, but how the patient copes with her incontinence should always be assessed; e.g. the size and type of pads worn may demonstrate how severe the incontinence is far more accurately than a description by the patient.

Drugs that Affect Incontinence

Class of drug	Effect on symptoms
Diuretics	Increased urgency, frequency, and urge incontinence
Some calcium antagonists	Urgency
Benzodiazepines	Sedation and confusion leading to secondary incontinence
Alcohol	Reduced mobility, diuresis, impaired perception of bladder filling, detrusor overactivity
Lithium	Urgency and frequency
Anticholinergics; e.g. antipsychotics, antidepressants, opiates, antispasmodics, and anti-Parkinsonian drugs	Impaired detrusor contractility causing urinary retention with overflow
Alpha blockers; e.g. doxazosin	Urinary incontinence due to urethral relaxation

Examination – What's Important
- Exclude an abdominal or pelvic mass
- Exclude full bladder
- Check for prolapse
- State of tissues
- Rough assessment of pelvic floor strength
- Neurological examination if indicated

Tackling Urinary Incontinence in Primary Care
- Exclude UTI
  - Urinalysis dipsticks are cheap and can exclude a UTI while the patient is in the surgery. An MSU can then be sent for culture and sensitivity on patients who are positive for nitrites and leucocytes on urine dipstick.
  - While a UTI may not be entirely responsible for a patient's incontinence, it can markedly exacerbate symptoms.

	Drink	Void	Leak
06:00			
07:00	150ml tea	200ml	
08:00		50ml	✓
09:00		50ml	
10:00			
11:00	150ml coffee	65ml	✓
12:00			✓
13:00	150ml tea		
14:00		100ml	
15:00			
16:00		30ml	
17:00		40ml	
18:00			
19:00	150ml tea	40ml	✓
20:00			✓
21:00			
22:00			
23:00	150ml tea		
00:00			
01:00		80ml	
02:00		100ml	✓
03:00			
04:00		50ml	
05:00			
Total:	900ml	795ml	

The Frequency/volume chart

Mrs JB*
51 years, widowed, lives alone

Symptoms
Urgency, frequency, nocturia, and urge incontinence

Frequency/volume chart findings
Fluid intake too little
All intake is caffeinated drinks
Only voiding small volumes

Action and advice
Exclude UTI and haematuria
Increase fluid intake to 1500–2000ml per day
Reduce tea and coffee to a maximum of three cups per day
Reduce fluid intake late at night
Repeat frequency/volume chart four weeks later to assess improvement

*this is a fictional example for the purposes of illustration

- Frequency/volume chart (see above)
  - Can show excessive drinking or bad habits.
- Appropriate fluid intake advice
  - Reduce caffeine-containing drinks; e.g. tea, coffee, and colas.
  - Increase water or berry juices, cranberry juice can be useful for reducing UTIs.
  - Appropriate amount; e.g. 1500-2500ml.
- Appropriate voiding habits
  - Double voiding.
  - Perineal hygiene; i.e. wiping from 'front to back' when bowels open.
  - Emptying the bladder before and after intercourse.
- Reducing coughing
  - Stopping smoking.
  - Optimising chest disease.

- Pelvic floor exercises
- Local oestrogen therapy (see p46)

Ideally, local guidelines for the management of patients with incontinence should be drawn up by a multidisciplinary team including PCGs, continence advisory services, district nurses, and urogynaecologists, so that the most effective use of the services can be achieved.

Although the definitive diagnosis usually needs to be made in secondary care, a caring and sympathetic approach to incontinence combined with an understanding of the embarrassment that these problems cause is invaluable in gaining a specific and honest history. The role of a sympathetic and supportive GP in broaching these sometimes difficult topics should not be underestimated.

When to refer and why

Bladder symptoms do not always correspond with urodynamic diagnosis and urgency in particular can be a symptom of many different conditions. A phrase that has been coined to describe this is 'the bladder as an unreliable witness'. This makes urodynamics important in assessing patients, particularly in those undergoing incontinence surgery.

Urodynamic diagnosis of patients presenting to primary care with the symptoms of stress incontinence:

- Urodynamic stress incontinence accounts only for 40–50% of symptomatic stress incontinence cases.
- Detrusor overactivity accounts for incontinence in 10–30% of these cases, while 30–40% actually suffer from mixed incontinence.

Other important causes of urgency
- *Urethral:* urethral syndrome, urethritis, urethral diverticulum
- *Bladder:* inflammation, infection, tumour, stone, radiotherapy
- *Gynaecological:* prolapse, pelvic mass, pregnancy, post-radical hysterectomy
- *Psychosomatic:* stress-induced, anxiety states
- *Neurological:* multiple sclerosis
- *Endocrine:* diabetes mellitus, myeloma
- *Iatrogenic:* diuretics

Anticholinergics can be prescribed before urodynamics in primary care for predominately irritative symptoms, providing any history of tumour, haematuria, or voiding difficulties have been excluded. Most gynaecologists, however, prefer to have a urodynamic diagnosis of detrusor instability before commencing these drugs.

Secondary Care Investigations
- Urinalysis/MSU
- Frequency/volume chart
  - Can show excessive drinking or bad habits.
  - Allows appropriate advice to be given.
- Uroflowmetry voiding
- Subtracted cystometry
- Video urodynamics is at present the gold standard but is only available in tertiary referral centres.
- Ambulatory urodynamics is also only available in tertiary referral centres. It has a high false positive rate and its role in clinical practice remains controversial.
- Pad test. Many different versions of the pad test exist. In the one-hour pad test the woman drinks 500ml of water and wears a pre-weighed sanitary towel for one hour, during which she performs some light exercise such as walking and stair climbing and some more provocative activities such as squats and hand washing. If the pad has gained more than 1g over the hour, this is suggestive of incontinence.

Urodynamics is cheap and relatively easy to perform, with district general hospitals usually able to offer subtracted cystometry. Voiding difficulties can be diagnosed (although the cause is not uncovered by urodynamics) and detrusor overactivity and urodynamic stress incontinence can be differentiated. Standard urodynamics is performed over 5-10 minutes and so only gives a snapshot of the behaviour of the detrusor muscle. This can pose problems; for example, a patient whose urgency is triggered by cold temperatures may find in a heated hospital room that her urodynamics are entirely normal.

What's Normal for the Female Bladder?
- Residual <50ml
- First sensation to void <250ml
- Cystometric bladder capacity 400–600ml
- Pressure rise of <10cm H_2O for 300ml
- Pressure rise of <15cm H_2O for 500ml
- No detrusor contractions during filling
- Maximum voiding pressure <60cm H_2O

Detrusor Overactivity and Treatment

Detrusor activity is the presence of spontaneous or provoked detrusor contractions during the filling phase when the patient is attempting to inhibit micturition. (ICS UK)

Detrusor overactivity is the second commonest cause of female urinary incontinence. The bladder should relax during filling but be able to contract during micturition. The cause of these overactive contractions is unknown, although suggestions include intrinsic overexcitability of the detrusor itself. It is usually idiopathic in origin, but detrusor overactivity may be linked to a lack of adequate bladder training as a child and emotional factors. It is becoming commoner as the population ages. Overactivity can also be secondary to upper motor neurone lesions, especially multiple sclerosis where it is known as detrusor hyperreflexia. Outflow obstruction is much rarer in women, but detrusor overactivity is seen after surgery for urodynamic stress incontinence secondary to partial obstruction of the urethra.

There are no physical signs with which to diagnose detrusor overactivity and the diagnosis must be made with urodynamics. To make diagnosis more challenging still, detrusor overactivity can be 'provoked' – coughing, sneezing, and laughing provoke large contractions in the detrusor and leakage. The patient may give a history that sounds like stress incontinence and it may even be demonstrated. The existence of provoked detrusor overactivity makes urodynamics essential, as the treatments for the two conditions are so different.

Drug treatment
Oestrogen
- Can reduce non-specific urinary tract symptoms in post-menopausal women, especially urgency, frequency, and dysuria
- Not effective in proven detrusor overactivity
- Topical vs systemic (see p46)

Oxybutinin
- Has anticholinergic and local anaesthetic effects
- Not specific for the bladder and has high rate of side-effects
- A long-acting 'XL' version is available with reduced side-effects

Tolterodine
- Relatively new antimuscarinic (side-effects include dry mouth, constipation, palpitations, blurred vision, drowsiness, heartburn, retention, dry skin, headache, paraesthesiae)
- Bladder specific
- As effective as oxybutinin with fewer side-effects
- 'XL' version with reduced side-effects available

Propiverine
- New bladder anti-spasmodic
- Market leader in Japan
- Acts as an anticholinergic and as a calcium channel blocker
- Has not yet been subject to trials against tolterodine or oxybutinin

Tri-cyclic antidepressants
- Anticholinergic effects and potentiate sympathetic bladder relaxation
- Have central sedative effects
- Can be very useful for nocturia
- Imipramine is longer acting with alpha adrenergic effects
- Amitriptyline is useful where bladder pain is an issue
- Side-effects include drowsiness or postural hypotension

Trospium chloride
- Anticholinergic
- Inert substance so has fewer drug interactions
- Does not cross the blood–brain barrier and so can be useful for patients who get headaches as a side-effect from more commonly used anticholinergics

Antidiuretic hormone analogues
- For example, synthetic vasopressin (DDAVP)
- Can now be used orally as well as intra-nasally
- Vasopressin is a peptide hormone that acts as a potent antidiuretic
- Has risk of hyponatraemia in elderly

Prescribing antimuscarinic drugs
Care needs to be taken, as antimuscarinics have many drug interactions. Risk of antimuscarinic side-effects are increased when taken with:
○ alcohol
○ some anti-arrhythmics
○ antidepressants; e.g. tricyclics and MAOIs
○ antihistamines
○ some antipsychotics; e.g. phenthiazine.

Anti-fungals – systemic absorption of ketoconazole is reduced.

Care with dopaminergics
○ Absorption of levodopa is reduced.
○ GI effects of metoclopramide and domperidone are increased.

Sub-lingual nitrate effects are reduced.

Behavioural therapy
During behavioural therapy patients relearn to inhibit a detrusor contraction. Options include:
- bladder drill
- biofeedback
- hypnotherapy.

Behavioural therapy and pharmacological treatment are a package and should be used together to achieve the optimum effect.

Bladder drill
Jarvis Regime
- Exclude pathology.
- Explain rationale to patient.
- The patient is given achievable set times to void; e.g. every 90 minutes and not allowed to void in between.
- When successful the voiding interval is increased; e.g. by 15–30 minutes.
- Maintain normal fluid intake of 1200–1500ml.
- Keep a fluid balance chart.
- Plenty of encouragement.

Bladder retraining can first be undertaken as an outpatient. Inpatient bladder training has a high success rate of up to 85% but unfortunately also has a high relapse rate when the women return to their normal environments and routines.

Difficulties with bladder retraining
- Time consuming, for both the woman and hospital staff.
- The patient needs to have a certain amount of intelligence and education to be able to understand the principles and fill in the fluid balance charts.
- The woman needs to be motivated.
- It does not work as well if undertaken more than once.

Biofeedback
Biofeedback is a technique where the patient is made aware of an autonomic function by using visual or auditory signals to demonstrate the strength of that autonomic function. Although good improvement rates can be achieved, biofeedback requires highly motivated staff with time to devote to it. It usually works best in specialist centres.

Hypnotherapy
One encouraging study has been performed using hypnotherapy to treat detrusor overactivity where 50% of the patients were symptom free after the course and 28%

reported an improvement in their symptoms. This study has never been substantiated by further work and each patient underwent 12 sessions in a four-week study period making it a time-consuming option.

Surgery for detrusor overactivity
Clam ileocystoplasty
Surgery is only performed for intractable severe detrusor overactivity. The operation most commonly performed is the 'clam ileocystoplasty' where the bladder is opened (like a clam) and a piece of ileum is sutured in like a patch. Complications include voiding difficulties, copious mucus production for the section of ileum, and a small risk of malignant change in the ileal segment.

Genuine Stress Incontinence and Treatment

Urodynamic stress incontinence:
Involuntary loss of urine when the intravesical pressure exceeds the maximum urethral closure pressure in the absence of detrusor overactivity. (ICS)

The bladder neck and the proximal urethra are usually intra-abdominal organs, above the pelvic floor and supported by the pubourethral ligaments. If either the pelvic floor muscles (the levator ani) or the pubourethral ligaments are damaged, the proximal urethra descends so that it is no longer an intra-abdominal organ. This makes the bladder neck weak, as it is no longer supported and leakage of urine occurs during stress such as coughing, laughing, sneezing, lifting, and bending. Stress incontinence is the commonest cause of female incontinence, accounting for about 50% of cases.

Conservative measures
Conservative treatment of stress incontinence should be used as first-line treatment, as they can often improve continence and do not cause harm. Conservative measures are particularly effective for:
  • mild stress incontinence
  • women who are medically unfit for surgery
  • women who want to avoid surgery
  • improving quality of life while waiting for definitive surgery
  • women who have not completed their family.

Physiotherapy
Vaginal cones
These are sets of five cones of increasing weight, usually 20-90g, that are inserted into the vagina. The woman contracts her pelvic floor muscles to prevent the cone from falling out.

The woman must have sufficient mobility and dexterity to be able to take the cones in and out. Women with prolapse are not always suitable, as the cones can lodge above the prolapse and not exercise the pelvic floor muscles. They are no more effective than well-supervised pelvic floor exercises.

Perineometry
This involves using a vaginal device to help assess the strength of contraction during pelvic floor exercises. It can help women to contract their pelvic floor muscles more appropriately and can also show improvements in the contraction strength. It can be used both in the hospital and by the woman at home.

Biofeedback (see p44)

Oestrogen
There is no evidence that oestrogen alone reduces stress incontinence. It may facilitate improvement when used in conjunction with other treatments and is important in subjective outcomes.

Topical vs systemic oestrogen therapy
Women, even on quite high systemic doses of HRT, can still have an atrophic lower genital tract. Local oestrogen may be more useful than systemic in treating lower urinary tract symptoms.

Types of local HRT
Creams and pessaries
For creams and pessaries patients need to have the mobility and dexterity to insert them. Some women find the pessaries less messy than the creams. The usual regimen is nightly for the first 14 days then twice-weekly maintenance. With this regimen there is no need to add in a progestogen. Ortho-Gynest products contain peanut oil and should not be given to women with peanut allergy!

Ring pessaries
These are softer and more flexible than the conventional rings used for replacing prolapse and last for three months before replacement is necessary.

Devices to aid continence
The continence devices have so far not made a great impact on management of stress incontinence. Robust data on their efficacy is lacking. Devices are either vaginal or urethral and maintain continence by occluding the urethra. These can only be used after specialist assessment and can be expensive.

Women with mild urodynamic stress incontinence can use a super plus variety of tampon to the same effect, as it lifts the bladder neck and causes a degree of outflow obstruction. Although evidence for this is anecdotal, some women find it useful to insert a tampon before exercise; e.g. before attending an aerobics class.

Most women with urodynamic stress incontinence need surgery and although conservative measures can be helpful, they often only cure women with mild symptoms.

Surgery
Surgery is usually the most effective way of curing urodynamic stress incontinence and up to a 90% cure rate can be achieved for an appropriate and well-performed primary repair. The aims of surgery are to:
- elevate the bladder neck, returning it to its rightful position as an intra-abdominal organ
- support the bladder neck behind the pubic symphysis
- increase outflow resistance
- stabilise the urethra.

Urodynamics is essential before surgery. Detrusor overactivity can be unmasked by surgery, as post-operatively the bladder contracts harder against the outflow obstruction created by the surgery. Detrusor overactivity can also arise *de novo* post-operatively and it is helpful for the surgeon to have documented evidence that the patient had a stable bladder pre-operatively. Urodynamics can also exclude pre-operative voiding difficulties and help choose patients suitable for surgery.

Surgical options
Of the many different operations, those currently of most importance are mentioned below.

Anterior colporrhaphy (anterior repair)
- There is little to commend anterior repair as a continence procedure. It has a poor success rate when compared with other continence procedures.

Marshall–Marchetti–Krantz (MMK)
- Does not treat cystocele.
- Now superseded by colposuspension/TVT.

Burch colposuspension
- Corrects stress incontinence and cystocele.
- Can perform a TAH at the same time if indicated.
- Ten years of follow-up data available.
- The role and success rates of laparoscopic colposuspension are still uncertain.

Tension-free vaginal tape
- Relatively new technique.
- Easy to perform with less time in hospital needed.
- Long-term follow-up data is lacking at present.
- Currently recommended procedure for urodynamic stress incontinence.

Injectables; e.g. macroplastique, GAX collagen
- Performed cystoscopically.
- Used to bulk up the bladder neck.
- Cure rates are 50% objective and 70% subjective after two years at best.
- New techniques and substances may become available to make this more successful.

The first operation that the patient undergoes has the greatest chance of success, so the decision of which operation is the best has to be taken on an individual basis and depends on many factors, such as fitness of the patient for anaesthetic and co-existing prolapse.

Artificial sphincter creation
- After conventional surgery fails.

Mixed Incontinence

Detrusor overactivity and stress incontinence can co-exist. This can be precipitated by, for example, a woman with stress incontinence who starts to try and keep her bladder empty to avoid leakage. The bladder then only becomes used to having very small amounts of urine in it and she gets symptoms of urgency when the bladder becomes fuller.

Voiding Difficulties

Voiding difficulties are a spectrum of disorders, including symptoms such as straining, hesitancy, and poor stream, through to acute or chronic retention.

Acute retention

A painful, palpable, or percussable bladder, when the patient is unable to pass any urine. (ICS)

Acute urinary retention can be a particular problem following labour and delivery with epidural or spinal analgesia, as in this situation urinary retention is painless and both the patient and midwife may be unaware of its existence. If this is left undiagnosed and untreated, it can result in long-term voiding difficulties.

Other causes of acute urinary retention
- Vulval herpes
- Bladder neck surgery

- Pelvic mass
- Urethral stenosis
- Foreign body in the urethra
- Retroverted gravid uterus

Chronic retention

A non-painful bladder which remains palpable or percussable after the patient has passed urine. Such patients may be incontinent. (ICS)

Chronic retention may be entirely asymptomatic or may present with frequency, overflow incontinence, and recurrent UTI.

Reasons for voiding difficulties
- *Failure of detrusor contraction.* This can be due to a neuropathy, old age, or if the bladder becomes very scarred.
- *Urethral pressure that is greater than the detrusor pressure.* This can be from bladder surgery such as an oedematous bladder neck, over-elevation during colposuspension, or a TVT pulled too tight. Other causes include urethral strictures or stenosis, urethral foreign bodies, or failure of the urethral sphincter to relax.
- *Detrusor sphincter dyssynergia.* This is where the urethral sphincter and the detrusor have lost their co-ordination, usually as part of a suprasacral cord lesion, and as the detrusor contracts, the urethra sphincter also contracts and urine remains in the bladder.

It is important to exclude neurological causes of voiding difficulties by performing a thorough neurological examination when these patients present. Neurological causes can be upper motor neurone, such as CVA, MS, or spinal cord trauma, or lower motor neurone, such as a prolapsed disc or a peripheral neuropathy.

Catheterisation is the mainstay of treatment for voiding difficulties. It empties the bladder and allows the detrusor to recover from overdistension. Definitive treatment depends on the underlying cause.

The Painful Bladder

There is a group of patients who suffer with urgency, frequency, nocturia, and a painful bladder despite UTI, detrusor overactivity, tumour, and calculi having been excluded. This collection of symptoms has been called sensory urgency, urgency-frequency syndrome, and interstitial cystitis. Other common features include an early first desire to void at urodynamics (<150ml) and a reduced cystometric bladder capacity (<300ml). Generally, the patients remain continent. It has been assumed that the symptoms are related to a chronic inflammation of the bladder, although the trigger or predisposing factors for this remain unclear. The mainstay of management is correct fluid intake and bladder drill. Drugs such as imipramine or tolterodine may also be useful.

Fistulae
Causes
- Congenital abnormalities (very rare)
- Avascular necrosis secondary to pelvic surgery
- Radiotherapy
- Malignancy
- Poor management of labour in the developing world causing ischaemic necrosis of the bladder base

Types
- Ureterovaginal
- Vesicovaginal
- Urethrovaginal
- Complex

Incontinence from fistulae is continuous, occurring day and night. The fistula is often visible on speculum. Surgical repair is usually required, although some vesicovaginal fistulae may heal with continuous bladder drainage and antibiotics.

Ongoing Care of the Incontinent Patient – Methods of Containment
Unfortunately, not all patients respond to treatment or are able to make the lifestyle adjustments necessary and a small but significant group of women will remain incontinent. It can be difficult for patients to obtain appropriate information on which incontinence products will be most suitable for their particular needs. Continence advisors and district nurses often have a wealth of knowledge and tips and can also provide emotional support to patients coming to terms with containment of their incontinence.

Pads
Because of the dearth of information available to them, women often use sanitary towels or a baby's nappies, which may be unsuitable.

Indwelling catheters
Long-term catheters are made from silicone and can be urethral or suprapubic and on free drainage or with a valve. Some elderly patients in particular may be more comfortable and dry with a catheter.

Clean intermittent self-catheterisation
Catheterisation empties the bladder and prevents overflow. The woman learns the

technique usually from a specialist nurse or continence advisor. For successful CISC the woman needs:

- motivation
- to find the technique acceptable
- adequate manual dexterity
- adequate mobility to be able to reach her urethra
- adequate mental awareness
- sufficient bladder capacity.

Different types of catheters are available, including self-lubricating, and it may take time to find the right product for the patient.

Urinary diversion

For a patient who is intractably incontinent, a bowel urinary diversion may be the most appropriate measure. The most common operation is an ileal conduit for which about 15–20cm of ileum is needed. Urinary diversion is most useful in young disabled patients.

Incontinence and the Elderly Patient

Elderly patients may only have the same level of incontinence as some younger women, but their ability to respond and compensate is impaired.

Causes of incontinence in the elderly woman

- Infection; e.g. UTI
- Confusional states; e.g. dementia or secondary to infection
- Faecal impaction
- Reduced mobility
- Depression
- Drug treatment; e.g. diuretics
- Endocrine disorders; e.g. diabetes
- Limited independence

Important differences in the incontinent elderly patient

- Maintain fluid intake at 2000–2500ml per day. The elderly are particularly susceptible to volume depletion because they have reduced total body water and increased body fat in comparison with younger adults. Reducing fluid intake below 2000ml per day may cause dehydration and confusion.
- Use anticholinergic medication with care. The elderly are more likely to have side-effects such as lethargy and confusion with anticholinergics.
- Nocturia may be a significant problem rather than incontinence in the day.
  A combination of factors makes nocturia a problem in the elderly patient:
  ○ The ability of the kidney to concentrate urine is decreased, so large volumes of dilute urine may be produced.

- ○ The glomerular filtration rate is increased in the supine position, so urine production increases when the patient lies down at night.
- ○ Delayed response to a fluid load with a nocturnal diuresis.
- ○ Loss of the diurnal variation in ADH, which normally suppresses urine production at night.
- ○ All of the above are increased further with pathology; e.g. CCF, diabetes mellitus, hypercalcaemia.

Other causes for nocturia, such as a poor sleep pattern, also need to be considered. Imipramine may be useful, improving both sleep and bladder function. Drugs for other conditions may exacerbate the elderly patient's incontinence:

- • *Diuretics.* Increase urinary frequency and urge incontinence.
- • *Calcium channel blockers.* Polyuria especially at night.
- • *Anticholinergics.* Confusion, especially if pre-existing confusion.
- • *a-adrenergic blockers.* Stress incontinence as they relax urethra.

Any sedative medication will increase continence problems.

Measures to help maintain continence in the elderly
- • Easy access to toilets
- • Appropriate rails and raised toilet seats
- • Easy to remove clothing – velcro fastenings; only one layer; short vests, blouses, and shirts that do not hang down

Some cognitively impaired patients may need prompted or scheduled toileting to maintain continence. However, this is labour intensive and carers may find it difficult to maintain.

Measures to reduce the impact of incontinence in the elderly
- • Wearing clothes made of easy-to-wash non-iron fabrics
- • Furniture protection – waterproof mattress; using waterproof draw sheets; waterproof covers for sofa cushions

Anal Incontinence

Involuntary loss of flatus, liquid or solid stool that is a social or hygienic problem.
(International Consultation on Incontinence)

Defining anal incontinence has been problematic and different definitions exist where flatus is not included or a minimum frequency of incontinent episodes has to be achieved. Although there are many causes for anal incontinence, patients with symptoms related to childbirth are those most frequently referred. Risk factors for anal incontinence are vaginal delivery, instrumental delivery, abnormal presentations, prolonged second stage, birth weight >4kg, and first baby.

Eighteen per cent of women will experience some faecal urgency after delivery and 10% will have had any faecal incontinence by three months postpartum. Fortunately, only a tiny percentage will have frank on-going incontinence of solid or liquid stool.

There is a considerable overlap between patients with urinary incontinence and those with faecal incontinence, with 20% of urogynaecological patients having some co-existing anal incontinence.

Ideally, women with childbirth-related anal incontinence should be assessed by a colorectal surgeon or gynaecologist with an interest in this area using anal physiology and endoanal ultrasound.

Treatment is either conservative, employing techniques such as physiotherapy, biofeedback, patient education, and altering stool consistency, or surgical, such as secondary overlapping anal sphincter repair.

Pelvic Organ Prolapse
Definitions
Cystocele: prolapse of the bladder and the anterior vaginal wall.
Rectocele: prolapse of the posterior vaginal wall and the rectum.
Uterine prolapse: descent of the uterus. This is divided into three degrees:
  • First degree: the uterus has moved down into the vagina but the cervix does not reach the introitus.
  • Second degree: the cervix is visible at the introitus.
  • Third degree or complete procidentia: the cervix and uterus are completely outside the vulva and vagina.
Enterocele: prolapse of the small bowel into the vagina often through the vault.
Vault prolapse: this usually describes prolapse of the vagina following hysterectomy.

More complex scoring systems exist so that the extent of prolapse can be identified and research studies can be standardised. These are not particularly useful tools in primary care and a basic but accurate description of the prolapse should be adequate for referral.

History and examination
Symptoms
  • Feeling of a lump in the vagina
  • Dragging sensation or lower backache
  • Symptoms associated with the site of the prolapse include cystocele (urinary frequency and urgency or retention) and rectocele (difficulty with evacuation of motions and digitation rectally or vaginally to empty the bowel)

Risk factors
- Parity (direct trauma during delivery and denervation injuries)
- Caucasian (prolapse is rare in Afro–Caribbean women)
- Smoking (coughing and effects on collagen)
- Postmenopausal
- Increased intra-abdominal pressure; e.g. persistent cough, heavy lifting, chronic constipation
- Steroids

Examination
- Exclude abdominal mass with PA and PV examination
- All newly diagnosed patients with prolapse should have an abdominal and pelvic ultrasound scan

Management
Conservative
- *Physiotherapy/pelvic floor exercises (see p45).*
- *Pessaries.* Many different pessaries have been manufactured over the years in a variety of different shapes, sizes, and materials. The patient should be reviewed every three to six months and the vagina examined with a speculum to exclude any ulceration.
- *Ring pessaries.* Ring pessaries sit behind the pubic symphysis pushing the vault posteriorly at the posterior fornix. Usually, a uterus is needed to be effective. Ring pessaries are often easy to change and although the assessment and initial fitting is typically performed in a hospital setting, many patients are subsequently successfully managed in the community.
- *Shelf pessaries.* These are occasionally used for vault prolapse. Generally, shelf pessaries are reviewed and changed in outpatients.

Who should have conservative management of prolapse?
○ Women unfit for surgery
○ Women not wanting surgery
○ Minor degree of prolapse
○ Women awaiting surgery

Some practitioners consider that conservative treatments should be tried with all patients, as they do little harm, may have significant benefit, and may enable the patient to understand which symptoms are related to their prolapse.

Surgical
Important points to bear in mind when discussing surgery:
- Continence problems should be excluded, as these can be masked by the prolapse.
- Ensure as far as possible that surgery addresses the patient's symptoms and concerns.
- Usually, sexual function is preserved with surgery, but the woman's expectations of sex after surgery should be discussed.
- Local HRT may improve tissues pre-operatively.

Patients need to know that prolapse surgery:
- may precipitate urinary incontinence
- has a 30% recurrence rate
- may alter the dynamics of the pelvic floor causing a different area to prolapse.

Many different operations have been described for reducing prolapse. Those most commonly used in clinical practice are:
- anterior repair to correct cystocele
- posterior repair to correct rectocele and/or enterocele and deficient perineum
- vaginal hysterectomy for uterine descent.

These operations are usually performed in combination depending on the patient's symptoms.

Operations to repair vault prolapse
- Sacrospinous fixation: the vaginal vault is secured to the sacral spines vaginally.
- Sacrospinous colpopexy: at laparotomy the vaginal vault is secured to the sacral spines using a synthetic mesh.

Useful tips
- Incontinence and prolapse, although benign conditions, significantly affect the patient's quality of life.
- With appropriate and sympathetic management in both primary and secondary care, quality of life can improve for almost all patients.
- New operative techniques and pharmacological approaches are being developed that offer considerable hope for patients in the future.

Further Reading

1. Maclean AB, Cardozo L (eds). *Incontinence in Women.* London: RCOG Press, 2002. The report of the 42nd RCOG Study Group.
2. Studd J (ed). *Progress in Obstetrics and Gynaecology.* Published by Churchill Livingstone, this is a series of books consisting of reviews of current interesting areas in the speciality. Several chapters are of particular interest to those wanting to know more about urogynaecology:
   - Jarvis GJ. Treatment of detrusor instability and urge incontinence. Vol. 14, 259-271.
   - Bidmead J, Cardozo L. Surgery for genuine stress incontinence. Vol. 14, 329-358.
   - Kozman EL, Frazer MI, Holland N. Uses of mechanical devices in the management of stress incontinence. Vol 13, 325-342.
3. Cardozo L, Staskin D, Kirby M. *Urinary Incontinence in Primary Care.* Plymouth: Isis Medical Media, 2000.
4. Hay-Smith EJC, Bø K, Berghmans LCM, *et al.* Pelvic floor muscle training for urinary incontinence in women (Cochrane Review). In: *The Cochrane Library,* Issue 4. Oxford: Update Software, 2002.
5. Thakar R, Stanton S. Management of urinary incontinence in women. *BMJ* 2000; **321:** 1326-1331.
6. Drug treatment of urinary incontinence in adults. *MeReC Bulletin* 2000; **11(3):** 9-12.
7. Thaker R, Stanton S. Management of genital prolapse. *BMJ* 2002; **324:** 1258-1262.
8. Abrams P, Cardozoh, Fall M, *et al.* The standardisation of terminology of lower urinary tract function: report from the standardisation sub-committee of the International Continence Society. *Neurology and Urodynamics* 2002: **21:** 167–178.

Useful Websites

- The International Continence Society UK has an annual multidisciplinary meeting largely devoted to clinical research into continence. They also have a website with links to other resources. URL: http://www.icsuk.org.uk.
- Incontact. 'A UK organisation for people affected by their bowel and bladder problems and their carers.' Offers information and support, helps with getting in touch with local services, provides regular newsletters, and gives the opportunity to meet others through the internet chatroom. United House, North Road, London N7 9DP. URL: http://www.incontact.org.uk.
- Bladder Pain Syndrome Association. C/o Winsley's House, High Street, Colchester CO10 1NG. URL: http://www.b-p-s-a.org.uk.

Screening and Cancers in Gynaecology

Dr Pallavi M Latthe, Mr Mahmood Shafi and Mr Santanu Baruah

Introduction

Breast cancer is by far the commonest cancer in women, accounting for nearly 30% of all new cases. Large bowel and lung cancer are respectively the second and third most common cancers in women. Ovarian and uterine cancer account for 5% and 4%, respectively, of the newly diagnosed cancers in females in the UK every year. However, the average GP sees only one new patient with ovarian cancer about every five years, and patients with other gynaecological cancers even less frequently.

Many women do not receive optimal diagnosis, assessment, or treatment. Undertreatment leads to reduced survival, while overtreatment is wasteful and causes avoidable adverse effects.

Screening for Cervical Cancer

Cervical cancer is the third commonest gynaecological cancer of female genital tract in the UK. Increasing the uptake of screening, alongside increasing informed choice, is of great importance in controlling this disease through prevention and early detection.

Pre-malignant disease of the cervix

The squamous and the columnar epithelium on the cervix meet at the SCJ. This junction moves according to hormonal stimulation throughout life. When columnar epithelium is exposed to the vaginal environment it changes into squamous epithelium through a process called metaplasia. This new metaplastic squamous epithelium under certain circumstances can give rise to various grades of abnormalities, including invasive cancer.

The pre-malignant condition of the cervix is called cervical intraepithelial neoplasia, a term first coined in 1960. This abnormality is confined to the cervical epithelium with an intact basement membrane. There are various nomenclatures to describe pre-malignant disease of the cervix.

There are three grades of CIN based on the depth of abnormality in the epithelium:
- CIN1: abnormality confined to the lower 1/3rd of epithelium

- CIN2: abnormality confined to the lower 2/3rd of epithelium
- CIN3: abnormality confined to the full thickness of epithelium.

HPV changes and CIN1 are also known as low-grade squamous intraepithelial lesion, while CIN2 and CIN3 are classified as high-grade squamous intraepithelial lesion. This classification system is also known as Bethesda system and a modified version of this is anticipated to be the standard nomenclature in the UK in near future.

CIN is asymptomatic and most of the low-grade lesions regress to normal without any treatment. 50% of the CIN lesions have potential to progress to invasive disease over 10–20 years. Up to 30% of the low-grade smears can appear as CIN3 on colposcopy.

Risk factors for cervical intraepithelial neoplasia and cervical cancer
- Multiple sexual partners
- HPV infection
- Presence of other genital neoplasia
- Smoking
- Presence of other STIs
- Immunodeficiency
- Previous CIN

NHS cervical screening programme
The NHSCSP was set up in 1988. Their computerised call and recall system keeps track of follow-up investigations and recalls women every three to five years, so it is important for all women to provide a correct name and address to their GP.

All women aged between 20–64 years are eligible for the cervical screening programme, which costs £132 million per year in England and Wales, or £34 per woman. Around 60% of health authorities invite women every three years and 15% have a mixed policy, inviting women every three or five years, depending on their age.

Women who have not had a recent smear test may be offered one when they attend their GP's surgery or family planning clinic on another matter. Women should receive their first invitation for routine screening before their 25th birthday.

In 2000–01, over four million women had a cervical smear, which covered 83% of the target population. Cervical smears every five years are expected to reduce cumulative incidence of cervical cancer by 80–90%.

How to take a cervical smear?
A cervical smear is taken from the SCJ with an Aylesbury spatula. The cervix is exposed with Cusco's speculum, then with firm even pressure and a 360 degree clockwise movement

the smear is taken from the SCJ. The sample should be spread onto a slide already labelled with the patient's details (name, date of birth, identification number, date of smear) in pencil and fixed immediately by flooding with a suitable cytological fixative. The fixative should be air-dried and the slide should be transported to the laboratory in a slide box to ensure that the smear is not damaged. All the details on the cervical smear request form should be meticulously filled to aid the interpretation of the slide by the cytologist.

Extended tip spatulas of various designs appear to be better for collecting endocervical cells than the commonly used Ayre spatula. The rate of detection of endocervical and metaplastic cells appears to be a valid and convenient surrogate for the ability to detect dyskaryosis and for adequate smear rates.

In day-to-day practice, a cyto brush is used in conjunction with a spatula in the following situations:
- the follow-up of previous endocervical glandular lesions (AIS or CGIN)
- pin point os at follow-up following treatment
- request from the laboratory.

To take a brush smear, insert the brush into the os, rotate clockwise, and spread on to a pre-labelled slide in a rolling motion. Ideally, spatula and brush smear should be applied to two different slides, but it may be applied to the same slide provided smears are labelled properly and not superimposed.

A problem-solving approach to smear taking
Atrophic cervix (e.g. after menopause)
- Use cytobrush.
- Moisten the Aylesbury spatula with normal saline before taking smear.
- Use local oestrogen cream two weeks prior to smear test.

Wide ectopy (e.g. Pill users)
- Sample from transformation zone, which is outside SCJ.
- Wipe the mucus if possible before smear taking.
- If it is reported as inadequate, then repeat in the first half of the cycle.

Purulent discharge (e.g. Candida, Chlamydia, Gardnerella, Trichomonas infection)
- Treat the infection first before taking smear.

Persistent cytolysis: (progesterone effect: second half of the cycle, Depo-Provera injection)
- Repeat smear before 10th day of the cycle.
- The hormonal effect cannot be avoided in case of exogenous hormones use.

Bleeding at smear taking: identify the cause
- Menstrual bleeding: defer smear-taking to next cycle.
- Vaginal infection: treat the cause.
- Any abnormal bleeding (post-coital, intermenstrual bleeding, postmenopausal bleeding): refer for further investigations.

Result of cervical smear
Cervical smears allow cytological analysis of the cells from the transformation zone by cytologists. Smear abnormalities are categorised as follows, depending on nuclear-cytoplasmic ratio, nuclear abnormality, or any other mitotic activity:
- BNA
- mild dyskaryosis
- moderate dyskaryosis
- severe dyskaryosis
- glandular abnormality.

Sometimes the smear is reported as 'unsatisfactory', which means that cells obtained for examination are not sufficient to give a diagnosis. The smears can be reported as unsatisfactory if the cells obtained are not from the SCJ (more common in postmenopausal women, those on combined pill, or pregnant women) or if the smear is mixed with blood (menstruating, cervical ectopy, cervical polyp).

Actions required for abnormal cervical smear results
- Unsatisfactory: repeat smear within three months
- BNA: repeat smear within six months, and in woman with persistent BNA (x 2) refer for colposcopy examination
- Mild dyskaryosis: as for BNA
- Moderate dyskaryosis: needs urgent referral for colposcopy examination
- Severe dyskaryosis: as for moderate dyskaryosis
- Glandular neoplasia or CGIN: as for moderate dyskaryosis

Once a referral is made an appointment in the colposcopy clinic is usually given by eight weeks in over 85% of cases; when referred for suspected malignancy the woman is seen within two weeks of referral.

Communicating results of the cervical smear to the women
Cervical screening is not a test to diagnose cancer. It is a test to check the health of the cervix. For one-in-ten women, the test shows changes in the cells that can be caused by many things. An abnormal cervical smear result can generate a significant amount of anxiety in patients. They need to be reassured that an abnormal cervical smear does not mean that they have cancer of the cervix. Smear is aimed to pick up pre-cancerous

abnormalities. Management of these abnormalities can prevent them from progressing into invasive cancer over 10–15 years.

Colposcopy and management of abnormal smear
Colposcopy is the examination of the cervix under microscope. To identify the abnormal epithelium, saline, 3% or 5% acetic acid, and Lugol's iodine are used. The lesions are graded according to various characteristics, like acetowhite areas, size and edge and definitions, iodine uptake, punctations, mosaicism, atypical vessels, and inter-capillary distance.

The management of any abnormality is dependent on patient age, size of the lesions, degree of abnormality, and availability of equipment. There are various procedures performed at a colposcopy clinic depending on indications, such as examination of the cervix, taking smear, punch biopsy, and excision or ablation of abnormal areas.

There are various techniques available for treatment of abnormal cervical epithelium:
- *Ablation methods.* Cryocautery, cold coagulation, radical electrodiathermy, and laser vapourisation.
- *Excisional methods.* Laser excision, LLETZ, and knife cone biopsy.

With excisional methods, the primary success rate is 95% (defined as negative smear in six months). LLETZ can be done under general anaesthesia, though it is usually performed under local anaesthesia. The result of the biopsy is usually communicated to the GP as well as to the patient as soon as it becomes available (two to four weeks).

The usual indications for treatment
- Moderate or severe dyskaryosis on smear
- High-grade lesion on colposcopy examination
- Glandular neoplasia
- Persistent low-grade abnormality

Follow-up care
Cytology is the mainstay, with colposcopy being optional at the first follow-up visit for early diagnosis of residual disease.

A typical follow-up protocol is as follows:
- first visit at six months at the colposcopy clinic for cytology and colposcopy
- annual visit from 12 months till five years at the GP's surgery for cytology.

Recent advances
Liquid-based cytology
In this alternative method, a smear is taken using either a plastic spatula or brush sampler to collect the cells from the cervix. The sample is then immediately transferred into a

preservative and sent to the laboratory. Smear takers find LBC simpler, convenient, and easy to use and there is a sharp reduction in the unsatisfactory smear rate, leading to less anxiety and discomfort for women. It results in more appropriate referrals to colposcopy; i.e. fewer unsatisfactory results and an improved detection rate of high-grade lesions of between three and nine women per 1000 tested. The residual LBC sample can be used for other tests where appropriate, such as HPV and Chlamydia, thus avoiding the need for separate examinations. LBC will help total automation of the screening programme. The ThinPrep Pap Test is now used in the Scottish Cervical Screening Programme.

Human papillomavirus testing
Human papillomavirus infection is important in the aetiology of cervical intraepithelial neoplasia. There are more than 70 subtypes of HPV available. The high-risk HPV subtypes are: 16, 18, 31, 33, and low-risk subtypes are 6 and 11. HPV 16 and 18 are present in 80% of cases of invasive cancer and 85% of high grade CIN. HPV 31 and 33 are responsible for the remainder. It is a sexually transmitted virus and causes transient and reversible cytological abnormality. In a minority of cases the infection persists and leads to cervical neoplasia. The various techniques available for detection of HPV are PCR, hybridisation, Southern blot, and Dot blot. Unfortunately, HPV screening in the general population is not a cost-effective option.

Cervical cancer
There were 2740 new cases of invasive cervical cancer in England and Wales in 1997. The NHSCSP claims successfully saving around 1300 lives per year, and being directly responsible for a 42% reduction in the incidence of cervical cancer between 1988 and 1997.

Who to refer
   • Women with moderate and severe dyskaryosis or malignant cells on cervical smear
   • Post-coital or intermenstrual bleeding
   • Postmenopausal bleeding
   • Offensive/bloodstained vaginal discharge
   • Abnormal appearance or texture of cervix

In cervical cancer, adequate pre-treatment assessment is vital. Surgery alone is sufficient for early cancers; radiotherapy is appropriate for later-stage cancers but is more likely to cause lasting adverse effects.

Simultaneous treatment with cisplatin and radiotherapy may increase survival rates in women with high-risk cervical cancer. Regular follow-up by gynaecological oncologists is then performed.

Endometrial cancer
Unlike cervical cancer, there is no endometrial cancer screening programme yet available. There are various risk factors attributed to the development of endometrial cancer, such as

age (peak incidence between 65–75 years), late menopause, nulliparity, obesity, unopposed oestrogen activity (HRT, Tamoxifen). There is a higher incidence of endometrial cancer among women with a personal or family history of cancer of ovary, breast, and colon. But none of these risk factors actually predicts the development of endometrial cancer.

The prognosis of endometrial cancer depends on early diagnosis and treatment. That is why early recourse to investigation for endometrial cancer is important.

Like cervical epithelium, endometrium has a pre-cancerous state called endometrial hyperplasia. There are three types: cystic, complex, and atypical hyperplasia. Both cystic and complex hyperplasia regress spontaneously in 90% of cases. Only 1–3% of cases progress to invasive disease. On the other hand, atypical endometrial hyperplasia can progress to invasive disease in 25% of cases. There may be co-existing cancerous changes in almost one-third of these cases. Hence, hysterectomy is recommended in such cases.

Both endometrial hyperplasia and endometrial cancer can present as: intermenstrual bleeding, vaginal discharge, polymenorrhoea in perimenopausal women, postmenopausal bleeding, pyometra, and glandular abnormalities on smear. Only a minority of cases of endometrial cancer (mostly in advanced stages) present with pelvic pain or uterine enlargement.

Patients with the following need referral
- Postmenopausal bleeding
- Abnormal cytology
- Postmenopausal vaginal discharge
- Menorrhagia, intermentstrual bleeding, or polymenorrhoea in perimenopausal women

Management in secondary care
Referrals for investigations for suspected endometrial cancer are seen within two weeks. The following modalities of investigations are carried out for investigation.

Hysteroscopy and curettage
It is performed as an inpatient or as an outpatient procedure. It allows the direct visualisation of the endometrium and sampling of the endometrium for histological diagnosis. Transvaginal ultrasound followed by outpatient biopsy offers rapid and accurate assessment.

Transvaginal ultrasound scan
Transvaginal ultrasound scan is aimed to assess the endometrium. Less than 4mm thickness of postmenopausal endometrium virtually excludes endometrial cancer. However, in the case of persistent bleeding, hysteroscopy and curettage is necessary.

Endometrial pipelle sampling
It is performed as an outpatient procedure, with the aim of getting endometrial cells for histological analysis. The sensitivity varies between 68–90%. Most women tolerate the procedure well.

Investigations for endometrial cancer reveal any of the three diagnoses: negative (i.e. normal endometrium), endometrial hyperplasia, and endometrial cancer. Those with negative diagnosis (95%) can be reassured and need no treatment.

Management of endometrial cancer
The mainstay of therapy is surgical. The disease is also staged based on findings at surgery and histology. Post-operative radiotherapy is indicated in the case of unfavourable pathology or if pelvic nodes are involved.

Ovarian cancer
Ovarian cancer has the highest mortality rate among all gynaecological cancers because it presents at a late stage (stage 3–4). It kills about 4000 women per year in England and Wales. The lifetime risk of developing ovarian cancer in the general population is 1.1%. Most of the ovarian cancers occur sporadically, but about 5% of ovarian cancers have genetic predisposition or are a part of the familial ovarian cancer. *BRCA1* gene mutation increases the lifetime risk of development of breast cancer by 85% and ovarian cancer by 60%. The other gene responsible for ovarian cancer development is a mutation of *BRCA2*. Lynch 2 gene-carrying families are at high risk of colorectal cancer (hereditary non-polyposis colorectal cancer), endometrial cancer, and ovarian cancer.

Protective effects against ovarian cancer
- COCP
- Pregnancy
- Breast feeding

Risk factors
- Family history of ovarian/breast/colon cancer
- Nulliparity
- Refractory involuntary infertility
- Age: rare before 30 years
- Social class 1 has twice the risk of class 5
- Causal relation with fertility drugs like clomiphene is not yet established, though there is some evidence of increased risk of borderline ovarian tumours after prolonged treatment with clomiphene

Those who have a personal or family history of ovarian/breast/colon cancer may be offered genetic counselling. The advantage of genetic counselling is that it can help to evaluate the lifetime risk of development of ovarian cancer, and if the risk is high prophylactic oophorectomy (once family is completed) can be offered. Screening women who are at risk because of a strong family history may be more cost effective, but this has not been established. Further evidence is required before a decision can be made concerning the potential benefits, harms, and costs of screening for ovarian cancer.

The methods available for detection for ovarian cancer are:
- tumour markers
- transvaginal ultrasound scan.

Tumour markers

CA125 is the most commonly used tumour marker for screening. Unfortunately, this marker is not specific. It is elevated in 82% of stage 3 and stage 4 epithelial ovarian cancers and in only 50% of stage 1 and stage 2 epithelial ovarian cancers.

CA125 can be raised in various benign conditions, such as endometriosis, PID, and even healthy women. It is also raised in non-gynaecological cancers (pancreas, stomach, colon, breast). Usually CA125 of more than 65IU/ml in premenopausal and 35IU/ml in postmenopausal women is an indication for further evaluation.

Other tumour markers, like CEA and CA19.9, help differentiate bowel and ovarian primary cancer. Alpha fetoprotein and hCG can be raised in sex cord stromal tumours.

Transvaginal ultrasound scan

Transvaginal ultrasound scan has the advantage of assessing the ovary and the pelvis. The use of colour Doppler has increased the sensitivity and specificity.

An ovarian volume over 20cm^3 in premenopausal woman or over 10cm^3 in postmenopausal woman is considered to be abnormal. The other markers for raising suspicion of malignancy are ascites, papillary projections, bilateral cysts, solid components, etc.

Morphologic indexing of the tumour is done along with CA125 and colour Doppler. The patient is then offered surgery if deemed necessary. It is important to make the woman aware that a negative test does not exclude the risk of development of ovarian cancer.

The following women should be referred to a gynaecological oncologist
- Abdominal distension, abdominal mass, pressure effect upon bladder/rectum with or without gastrointestinal symptoms or/and sudden weight loss.
- Those who have a strong family history of breast/ovary/endometrium/colon cancer (two or more close relatives).
- Any ovarian cyst diagnosed accidentally on USS in postmenopausal women.

Management of ovarian cancer in secondary care

The primary surgery for advanced ovarian cancer is total abdominal hysterectomy, bilateral salpingo-oophorectomy, omentectomy, and peritoneal washings with pelvic and para-aortic lymph node sampling or removal. The aim of surgery is to remove all macroscopic deposits. It is not always possible to perform a complete de-bulking surgery for advanced stage carcinoma of the ovary. Chemotherapy should be considered in most ovarian cancer cases apart from stage 1a. Simple oophorectomy may be an indication in the case of young women (where fertility is an issue) in stage 1a with favourable histology.

Useful tips

○ Though the onset of symptoms is insidious in most women, ovarian cancer can occasionally present with acute onset of pelvic pain when the cyst undergoes torsion, haemorrhage, or rupture.
○ Women with ovarian cancer live longer if expert multidisciplinary teams treat them, and if gynaecological oncologists carry out surgery.
○ Chemotherapy can extend the lives of women with advanced ovarian cancer. Current evidence suggests that the optimal treatment is with paclitaxel/carboplatin.

Vaginal cancer

Vaginal invasive cancer and VaIN are poorly characterised and commoner in women with other lower genital tract preinvasive disease, like CIN. Both these conditions are managed in a large centre where expertise in gynaecologic oncology and radiotherapy is available. Any woman with abnormal vaginal bleeding, discharge, or vaginal growth should be referred promptly.

Vulval preinvasive and invasive disease

Vulval preinvasive disease commonly is squamous VIN and rarely it can present as Paget's disease or melanoma in-situ.

Who to refer

• Women with pruritus, burning pain/soreness not responding to standard treatment.
• Women with raised or flat, leucoplakia, ulceration, reddened hyperkeratotic, pigmented lesions on the vulva.

The malignant potential of VIN is unknown. In most hospitals, the mainstay of the treatment is local excision of the symptomatic areas, but it can recur, especially in younger women and in those with multifocal disease. Lichen sclerosus is known to have a definite malignant potential.

Vulval cancer is a heterogenous and uncommon condition. Multidisciplinary teams in the cancer centres are involved in the management of vulval cancer. It can range from wide local excision to radical vulvectomy with bilateral groin node dissection. Rarely, antero-posterior resection may be carried out, though chemo-radiotherapy is more commonly given in the advanced stages or for recurrent disease.

Further Reading

1. University of York. NHS Centre for Reviews and Dissemination. The management of gynaecological cancers. *Effective Health Care* 1999; **5(3):** 1–12.
2. Teale G, Jordan JA. Lower genital tract intraepithelial neoplasia. In: Shafi MI, Luesley DM, Jordan JA (eds). *Handbook of Gynaecological Oncology.* [1st ed.] Edinburgh: Churchill Livingstone, 2001; 151–166.
3. Martin-Hirsch P, Jarvis G, Kitchener H, Lilford R. Collection devices for obtaining cervical cytology samples (Cochrane Review). In: *The Cochrane Library,* Issue 3. Oxford: Update Software, 2002.
4. Shafi MI. Conservative management of CIN. In: Luesley DM, Shafi MI, Jordan JA (eds). *Handbook of Colposcopy.* [2nd ed.] London: Arnold, 2002; 88–94.
5. Shafi MI. Cervical cancer. In: Shafi MI, Luesley DM, Jordan JA (eds). *Handbook of Gynaecological Oncology.* [1st ed.] Edinburgh: Churchill Livingstone, 2001; 201–214.
6. Martin-Hirsch P, Reynolds K. Endometrial cancer. In: Shafi MI, Luesley DM, Jordan JA (eds). *Handbook of Gynaecological Oncology.* [1st ed.] Edinburgh: Churchill Livingstone, 2001; 215–230.
7. Bell R, Petticrew M, Luengo S, Sheldon TA. Screening for ovarian cancer: a systematic review. *Health Technol Assess* 1998; **2(2):** 1–84.
8. Acheson N, Chan KK. Epithelial ovarian cancer. In: Shafi MI, Luesley DM, Jordan JA (eds). *Handbook of Gynaecological Oncology.* [1st ed.] Edinburgh: Churchill Livingstone, 2001; 231–242.
9. Ind T. Management of postmenopausal bleeding. In: Studd J (ed). *Progress in Obstetrics and Gynaecology.* [Vol. 13.] London: Churchill Livingstone, 1998; 361–378.
10. Luesley DM (ed). Standards and Quality in Colposcopy. NHSCSP Publication, 1996.
11. Austoker J, Davey C (eds). Cervical smear results explained: a guide to primary care. NHSCSP Publication, 1997.
12. National Institute of Clinical Excellence. Guidelines on the use of liquid-based cytology for cervical screening. June, 2001.

Useful Websites

- NHS Cervical Screening Programme (NHSCSP).
  URL: http://www.cancerscreening.nhs.uk/ cervical/index.html.
- The British Society for Colposcopy and Cervical Pathology (BSCCP).
  URL: www.bsccp.org.uk.
- iNHiS guide to cancer information.
  URL: http://www.inhis.nhs.uk/Cancer/gynaecological_ cancer_home.htm.

Pelvic Infections and Vaginitis

Dr Manish Latthe, Dr Pallavi M Latthe and Dr Sirjit S Bath

Introduction
In this chapter we will discuss some of the common gynaecological infections that present to GPs, including pelvic inflammatory disease and vaginal discharge.

Pelvic Inflammatory Disease
Pelvic inflammatory disease is inflammation of the upper genital tract in women, typically involving the Fallopian tubes, ovaries, and surrounding structures.

About 20% of affected women become infertile, 20% develop CPP, and 10% of those who conceive have an ectopic pregnancy. Repeated episodes of PID are associated with a four-to-six-fold increase in the risk of permanent tubal damage. Therefore, diagnosis and treatment must be prompt.

The incidence is about 10–12 cases per 1000 women of reproductive age (about 8–10% of sexually active women in the UK are thought to be infected). However, exact incidence and prevalence are difficult to determine, as many cases of PID are asymptomatic.

Risk factors for acute pelvic inflammatory disease
- Age below 35 years (between 16–19 years for Chlamydia)
- Multiple sexual partners or recent new partner
- Previous PID
- Use of an intra-uterine contraceptive device
- Presence of bacterial vaginosis or an STI
- Nulliparity
- Recent instrumentation of the uterus (e.g. termination of pregnancy)
- African or Afro-Caribbean ethnic origin

PID results from a number of organisms both aerobic and anaerobic. *Neisseria gonorrhoeae* is the most common cause of PID. *N. gonorrhoeae* can also cause sepsis, migratory polyarthritis, endocarditis, anal infection, and urethritis; the last may be asymptomatic in women. Male-to-female is the commonest route of transmission.

Another cause is Chlamydia. *Chlamydia trachomatis* has 15 serotypes, which cause a range of infections from Bartholin's gland infection to conjunctivitis and oropharyngeal infections, and infects about 5% of non-pregnant women. The most common clinical infection due to Chlamydia is cervicitis. Up to 70% of women with an infection are asymptomatic in the early stages, but they can still pass the disease on to a partner. The incubation period for men is between one and three weeks, but up to 50% of them will be asymptomatic as well. (Once symptoms appear, they usually persist. In some cases, they may only last a few days and then disappear again, but the infection may still be present.) Genital Chlamydia is the most common curable STI in the UK. The doctor should be alerted to the possibility of Chlamydia in any woman presenting with irregular periods, spotting, dyspareunia, pelvic pain, or discharge.

Occasionally anaerobes (including bacteroids and anaerobic cocci), Gram-negative aerobic rods, and Gram-positive aerobes (including group B Streptococcus) can lead to acute PID.

Symptoms and signs
Patients usually present with pelvic pain associated with a temperature and vaginal discharge. There may be some systemic symptoms. Particularly in the case of Chlamydia, there may just be abnormal bleeding or post-coital bleeding.

Clinical criteria represent the best diagnostic method for discriminating PID from other infections. The woman commonly presents with symptoms frequently occurring during or after menses:
  • lower abdominal pain
  • fever
  • nausea and vomiting
  • vaginal discharge
  • intermenstrual bleeding or post-coital bleeding.

Examination findings
  • Pyrexia and tachycardia are present, often with signs of dehydration if the patient has vomiting.
  • Abdominal tenderness with or without rebound tenderness is caused by peritoneal irritation.
  • Cervix appears red and bleeds easily when touched; yellow-green mucopurulent discharge might be visible.
  • Bilateral lower abdominal tenderness with guarding, rebound tenderness, and cervical motion tenderness can be elicited.

N. gonorrhoeae infection is usually more acute than Chlamydia, with a more rapid onset. Pelvic pain develops shortly after menses starts and although the pain is often localised to one side, both tubes are usually infected. Peritonitis may occur, causing upper abdominal pain and adhesions. Chlamydial infections are milder but can cause more damage than *N. gonorrhoeae* in the long term.

Diagnosis
Minimum clinical criteria to institute empirical treatment of PID
- Lower abdominal tenderness
- Adnexal tenderness
- Cervical motion tenderness

Additional criteria
- Increase the specificity of diagnosis

Routine criteria
- Oral temperature >38.3° C (>100.9° F)
- Abnormal cervical or vaginal discharge
- Elevated ESR
- Elevated C-reactive protein
- Laboratory documentation of cervical infection due to *N. gonorrhoeae* or *C. trachomatis* by endocervical swabs

Elaborate criteria
- Histopathologic evidence of endometritis on endometrial biopsy
- Tubo-ovarian abscess on ultrasound scan or other radiological tests
- Laparoscopic abnormalities consistent with PID

Raised white cell count is typical. In males, Chlamydia and gonorrhoea are detected in the urethral discharge, which is done by taking a urethral swab. It is also possible to detect Chlamydia by analysing the urine sample using PCR.

Differential diagnosis includes ectopic pregnancy, acute appendicitis, endometriosis, symptomatic ovarian rupture, ovarian neoplasm, and uterine fibroids. Vaginal foreign bodies (e.g. lost tampons) may also cause similar symptoms and toxic shock syndrome must not be overlooked.

Treatment
Uncomplicated gonorrhoea
Single-dose treatment with ciprofloxacin or ofloxacin or cefotaxime in uncomplicated infection is sufficient.

Uncomplicated genital chlamydial infection, non-gonococcal urethritis, and non-specific genital infection
Treat with doxycycline for seven days or with azithromycin as a single dose; alternatively, treat with erythromycin for 14 days.

Pelvic inflammatory disease
Treat for at least 14 days; in severely ill patients substitute initial treatment with doxycycline + cefoxitin, then switch to oral treatment with doxycycline + metronidazole to complete 14 days' treatment; remember to treat for gonorrhoea.

When to refer

Useful tips
Criteria for hospitalisation for patients with acute PID
○ The diagnosis is uncertain, and surgical emergencies like appendicitis and ectopic pregnancy cannot be excluded.
○ Pelvic abscess is suspected.
○ Patient is pregnant.
○ Patient is adolescent (unpredictable compliance).
○ The patient has HIV infection.
○ Severe pain, nausea, vomiting preclude treatment at home.
○ The patient is unable to tolerate or has failed to respond to outpatient therapy.

Complications needing referral to secondary care
- Chronic salpingitis can be diagnosed by tubal scarring and adhesion formation on laparoscopy; long-term consequences include CPP, menstrual irregularities, and infertility.
- Tubo-ovarian abscess develops in about 15% of women with salpingitis. It can accompany acute or chronic infection and may require prolonged hospitalisation, sometimes with surgical drainage. Rupture of the abscess is a surgical emergency, with symptoms such as severe lower abdominal pain, nausea, vomiting, generalised peritonitis, and septic shock.
- Pyosalpinx (one or both Fallopian tubes filled with pus) may also be present. The fluid may be sterile, but leucocytes predominate in it.
- Hydrosalpinx (fimbrial obstruction and tubal distention with non-purulent fluid) develops if treatment is late or incomplete. The consequent mucosal destruction leads to infertility. Hydrosalpinx is generally asymptomatic but can cause pelvic pressure, CPP, or dyspareunia.
- Fitz–Hugh–Curtis syndrome can be a complication of gonococcal or Chlamydial salpingitis. It is characterised by right upper quadrant pain in association with acute salpingitis, indicating perihepatitis. Acute cholecystitis may be suspected, but symptoms and signs of PID are present or develop rapidly.

Management in secondary care
- Pelvic ultrasonography is done when a patient cannot be adequately examined because of tenderness or pain, when a pelvic mass may be present, or when no response to antibiotic therapy occurs within 48–72 hours.

- Intravenous antibiotic therapy is commenced if there is no response to oral antibiotics in 24–36 hours.
- Symptomatic and supportive treatment with anti-emetics, analgesics, and intravenous fluids is given.
- Diagnostic laparoscopy is the first step to diagnose complications due to PID. Laparoscopy has the best specificity, and is thus useful in those cases progressing with an atypical clinical course for discarding abdominal pain caused by another factor. Laparoscopic management can include adhesiolysis, salpingectomy, oophorectomy, tuboplasty, and drainage of abscess.
- In cases of long-term PID with symptoms, pelvic clearance in the form of total abdominal hysterectomy and bilateral salpingo-oophorectomy can be offered.

Management of Chlamydia positive cases
- There are various regimes available for treatment for Chlamydia infection, as stated above. Azithromycin 1g single dose, doxycycline 100mg twice daily, or erythromycin 500mg thrice daily for seven days are equally effective.
- All Chlamydia positive cases should be referred to a GUM clinic. GUM clinics organise contact tracing as well as treatment for the sexual partner(s).

Prevention of pelvic inflammatory disease
- Condoms prevent transmission of STIs from male to female, including HIV and hepatitis B. There is good evidence that the spermicide nonoxynol-9 does not protect against STIs, and there is some evidence that it may be harmful by increasing the rate of genital ulceration. As such, this product cannot be recommended for STI prevention.
- The use of oral contraceptive pills is known to reduce the risk of developing acute PID.
- Contact tracing and treatment of infected partners.

C. trachomatis *screening*
There is evidence to support a level B recommendation (based on robust experimental or observational studies) that screening for Chlamydia using culture is effective in preventing PID in the short term. As yet, there is no consensus as to whether there is enough evidence to implement a population-based screening programme as opposed to an opportunistic one. Endocervical swab and first voided urine can be collected for screening for Chlamydia. Nucleic acid amplification tests, which use non-invasive samples such as urine, are more effective at detecting asymptomatic chlamydial infection than conventional tests, but there are few data to relate a positive result with clinical outcome.

It is important to learn how to take endo-cervical swabs correctly to diagnose Chlamydia. One study estimated that 10–35% of endo-cervical swabs are performed inadequately.

Tips for collection of endo-cervical swab
- Explain the procedure to the patient.
- View the cervix with Cusco's speculum and remove any mucus and vaginal secretions.
- Insert a sterile cotton tip swab 1–2cm into the endo-cervical canal and rotate.
- Rotate the tip for 20–30 seconds and withdraw.
- Directly place in the transport medium.

Vulvovaginal Infections
Bacterial vaginosis
A patient with bacterial vaginosis, the most common cause of abnormal vaginal discharge, usually presents with a persistent smelly vaginal discharge. Although bacterial vaginosis is usually diagnosed in sexually active women (10–40% prevalence) and is present with other STIs, it has not been proven to be sexually transmitted and can occur without sexual activity. It results from the loss of the normal hydrogen peroxide-producing lactobacilli and an increase in the numbers of mycoplasma, Gardnerella, mobiluncus species, and anaerobic bacteria. There is no inflammation of the vaginal epithelium, hence the term vaginosis as opposed to vaginitis.

Diagnosis
- Homogenous white discharge and an unpleasant (fishy) odour.
- Microscopic examination of a slide from high vaginal swab will reveal 'clue cells'.
- A 'whiff test' can be conducted, in which a drop of vaginal discharge is placed on the slide and a drop of 10% potassium hydroxide is added. If anaerobic bacteria are present, a fishy odour of amines will be noted.
- A pH level greater than 4.5 of the vaginal discharge will be indicative of bacterial vaginosis.

Treatment of bacterial vaginosis

First line
○ Metronidazole 400mg twice daily for seven days

Alternative regimens
○ Clindamycin cream 2%, one full applicator intravaginally at bed time for seven days
○ Clindamycin 300mg twice daily orally for seven days
○ Metronidazole 2g orally single dose

Pregnant patients
○ Metronidazole is contraindicated in the first trimester; clindamycin cream or metronidazole gel is preferred in 2nd or 3rd trimester

Treatment of the partner does not reduce recurrence. Even though treatment clears the symptoms, recurrence is common, as it takes several weeks for the normal flora of the vagina to return. Treatment of asymptomatic patients remains unclear and is the subject of ongoing studies.

Candidiasis
This is the commonest cause of pruritic vaginal discharge. It is usually due to infection with *Candida albicans*.

Diagnosis
- High risk groups: diabetes, Cushing's or Addison's disease, pregnancy, and women who wear tight clothing. Higher incidence is noted in women taking certain drugs like antibiotics/steroids/combined pill/immunosuppressants.
- This usually presents with a thick white discharge associated with pruritus.
- There may be erythema of the vagina and vulva.
- Diagnosis is confirmed by a high vaginal swab microscopy and culture.

Treatment of symptomatic vulvovaginal candidiasis in non-pregnant women
- Intravaginal imidazoles (e.g. clotrimazole) significantly reduce persistent symptoms of vulvovaginal candidiasis after one month; NNT: 3.
- There is no clear evidence that effects differ significantly among the various intravaginal imidazoles. No difference between shorter and longer durations of treatment (1–14 days).
- RCTs have found no significant difference in persistent symptoms with oral fluconazole, ketoconazole, or itraconazole versus intravaginal imidazoles.
- Intravaginal nystatin: one RCT found that intravaginal nystatin significantly reduced the proportion of women with a poor symptomatic response after one week; NNT: 3.
- Fluconazole is associated with increased frequency of mild nausea, headache, and abdominal pain.
- There is no clear evidence that treating a woman's male sexual partner significantly improves resolution of the woman's symptoms or reduces the rate of symptomatic relapse.

Prophylaxis
- *Oral itraconazole.* One RCT found that oral itraconazole significantly reduced recurrence over six months; NNT: 4.
- *Prophylaxis with intermittent or continuous ketoconazole.* One RCT found that oral ketoconazole (given either intermittently or continuously at a lower dose) versus placebo significantly reduced symptomatic recurrences over six months; NNT: 2–4.
- *Regular prophylaxis with oral fluconazole.* There are no RCTs about the effects of fluconazole in preventing recurrence of vulvovaginal candidiasis.

- *Regular prophylaxis with intravaginal imidazole.* RCTs comparing regular prophylaxis with intravaginal imidazole versus placebo found inconsistent effects on the proportion of women with symptomatic relapse. One RCT found that regular prophylactic intravaginal imidazole versus treatment at the onset of symptoms reduced the frequency of episodes of symptomatic vaginitis, but the difference was not significant. The RCTs were too small to exclude a clinically important benefit.

Pregnant patients
- Topical therapies only, seven-day regimen (clotrimazole, miconazole, terconazole, butoconazole, and nystatin).

Complementary therapy for bacterial vaginosis and candidiasis
The available evidence for alternative treatments of vaginitis is of poor quality despite the prevalent use of these therapies.
- Lactobacillus recolonisation (via yoghurt or capsules) shows promise for the treatment of both yeast vaginitis and bacterial vaginosis with little potential for harm.
- Boric acid can be recommended for recurrent vulvovaginal candidiasis if resistance to conventional therapies is encountered but can occasionally cause vaginal burning.
- Because of associated risks in the absence of well-documented clinical benefits, douching should not be recommended.
- Finally, tea tree oil and garlic show some in vitro potential for the treatment of vaginitis, but the lack of in vivo studies precludes their recommendation to patients for the time being.

Trichomoniasis

This infection caused by the flagellated protozoan *Trichomonas vaginalis* is particularly prevalent in women with multiple sexual partners and is an STI. Infection can lead to abnormal cervical smears, which should be repeated after eradication therapy.

Presentation can vary widely from absence of symptoms to severe itching/burning and dyspareunia. Occasionally, dysuria is present. There is usually a frothy vaginal discharge, which may be green or yellow-grey. The cervix may look ecchymosed, or 'like strawberry'. The vaginal skin is reddish purple and swollen but not as red as candidiasis. A high vaginal swab (fresh wet mount of mobile flagellated organisms) will confirm the diagnosis.

Treatment is effected by metronidazole 400mg twice daily for seven days or 2g as a single dose orally to both partners. After the first trimester, pregnant patients may be treated with 2g metronidazole in a single oral dose. Referral to a local GUM clinic will enable contact tracing and screening for other STIs.

Herpes simplex virus

Humans are the only natural reservoir for HSV. Transmission is through direct contact with infected secretions via mucocutaneous sites of cut or diseased skin. Transmission occurs both from people with active lesions and asymptomatic excretors. HSV type 2 causes 70% of herpetic genital tract infections. When it is transmitted sexually the highest rate of infection is between 15 and 25 years of age.

Patients usually present with painful vulval and vaginal ulcers associated with discharge and dysuria. There may also be systemic signs. About 70% of cases will have recurrent mucosal lesions and periods of asymptomatic shedding within the first year of primary infection.

Treatment is with oral antiviral drugs acyclovir, famciclovir, or valiciclovir for five days. For recurrent infection higher doses may be needed. Oral analgesia (non-steroidal anti-inflammatory agents) will be required for acute lesions. Sufferers of repeated severe infections (more than six a year) may need prophylaxis. Sexual counselling will also be needed and is usually offered through the local GUM clinic.

If the woman is infected for the first time in pregnancy, she is treated with oral acyclovir. If there are active lesions at the time of childbirth, caesarean section may be recommended to prevent transmission to the newborn baby.

Human papillomavirus

Human papillomavirus has been strongly implicated as a cause of cervical cancer as with many other ano-genital cancers. Some papillomavirus infections cause no epithelial change and others cause cervical warts. These are usually asymptomatic but can be seen as white patches at colposcopy with the application of acetic acid. Cervical smears from women with these warts are usually reported as 'dyskaryosis' or 'CIN'.

HPV infection is commonest in women in their 20's. It is unknown why infection persists in some women and goes on to develop malignant cervical changes. Theories include intensity of infection, age at exposure, genital hygiene, immune response, or reproductive history. Most changes seem to be reversible and lesions of different severity seem to co-exist in the same patient.

At present active treatment is not recommended, but regular smears are suggested. HPV subtyping at cervical smears is useful in assessing the extent of treatment and intensity of surveillance. Vaccines have been developed against HPV and are being evaluated in clinical trials.

Useful tips

- ○ Use of laboratory diagnosis is essential.
- ○ Chlamydia is commonly asymptomatic.
- ○ Contact tracing is important and recommended in all STIs.
- ○ Severe infections need hospital treatment.
- ○ The risk of IUD-associated infection is low, with or without use of antibiotic prophylaxis.
- ○ There is no difference between the relative effectiveness of oral and intravaginal anti-fungal treatment for thrush.
- ○ Don't forget about the possibility of foreign bodies as a cause of discharge; e.g. tampons.

Further Reading

1. Ross J. Pelvic inflammatory disease. *BMJ* 2001; **322**: 658-659.
2. Hicks NR, Dawes M, Fleminger M, *et al.* Evidence based case report: chlamydia infection in general practice. *BMJ* 1999; **318**: 790-792.
3. Duncan B, Hart G, Scoular A, Bigrigg A. Qualitative analysis of psychosocial impact of diagnosis of Chlamydia trachomatis: implications for screening. *BMJ* 2001; **322**: 195-199.
4. Santer M, Warner P, Wyke S, Sutherland S. Opportunistic screening for chlamydia infection in general practice: can we reach young women? *J Med Screen* 2000; **7**: 175-176.
5. Brocklehurst P, Rooney G. Interventions for treating genital chlamydia trachomatis infection in pregnancy (Cochrane Review). In: *The Cochrane Library*, Issue 1. Oxford: Update Software, 2003.
6. Watson MC, Grimshaw JM, Bond CM, *et al.* Oral versus intra-vaginal imidazole and triazole anti-fungal treatment of uncomplicated vulvovaginal candidiasis (thrush) (Cochrane Review). In: *The Cochrane Library*, Issue 1. Oxford: Update Software, 2003.
7. ClaSS Study Group. Evidence is not (yet) enough for evidence based policy for chlamydia screening. *BMJ* 2001; **322**: 364.
8. Marrazzo J. Vulvovaginal candidiasis. *BMJ* 2002; **325**: 586.
9. Langsford MJ, Dobbs FF, Morrison GM, Dance DA. The effect of introduction of a guideline on the management of vaginal discharge and in particular bacterial vaginosis in primary care. *Fam Pract* 2001; **18**: 253-257.
10. Watson EJ, Templeton A, Russell I, *et al.* The accuracy and efficacy of screening tests for Chlamydia trachomatis: a systematic review. *J Med Microbiol* 2002; **51**: 1021-1031.
11. Van Kessel K, Assefi N, Marrazzo J, Eckert L. Common complementary and alternative therapies for yeast vaginitis and bacterial vaginosis: a systematic review. *Obstet Gynecol Surv* 2003; **58**: 351-358.

12. Watson MC, Grimshaw JM, Bond CM, *et al*. Oral versus intra-vaginal imidazole and triazole anti-fungal agents for the treatment of uncomplicated vulvovaginal candidiasis (thrush): a systematic review. *BJOG* 2002; **109:** 85-95.

Useful Websites

- Chlamydiae.com is a website providing information for both patients and health care professionals about this infection. URL: http://www.chlamydiae.com/chlamydiae/.
- Women's Health. URL: http://www.womenshealthlondon.org.uk/.
- Playingsafely.com. URL: http://www.playingsafely.co.uk.
- Society of Health Advisors in Sexually Transmitted Diseases.
  URL: http://www.shastd.org.uk/.

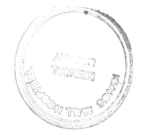

Pelvic Pain

Dr Swati Jha

Introduction

Pelvic pain is one of the most common causes of gynaecological referrals and has a major impact on work productivity and health care utilisation. Pelvic pain may be acute or chronic. Whereas acute pelvic pain tends to present as an emergency, chronic pelvic pain can be a cause of considerable physical discomfort as well as psychosocial upheaval.

Some commonly used terms in relation to pelvic pain are as follows:
- *Acute pelvic pain.* Pelvic pain of sudden onset.
- *Chronic pelvic pain.* Pelvic pain of more than six months' duration.
- *Dysmenorrhoea.* Painful menstruation, which may be primary or secondary. Primary dysmenorrhoea applies to women with no pathological cause, and secondary dysmenorrhoea applies to women with a pathological condition causing the dysmenorrhoea.
- *Dyspareunia.* Painful intercourse.
- *Dyschezia.* Painful bowel movement.

Acute Pelvic Pain
Aetiology
Pregnancy related
- Miscarriage (threatened, incomplete, inevitable septic; 1-in-5 pregnancies)
- Ectopic pregnancy (1-in-200 pregnancies)
- Rupture of a corpus luteum cyst
- Pre-term labour (7% of pregnancies)
- Abruptio placentae (0.4–3.5% of pregnancies)
- Uterine rupture or scar dehiscence (uncommon; 2 per 1000)

Gynaecological
- Primary dysmenorrhoea
- Acute PID
- Mittelschmerz (ovulation pain)
- Ovarian cyst accident (haemorrhage, rupture, or torsion)
- Degenerative changes in fibroids

- Pelvic neoplasm
- Acute pelvic vein thrombosis

Miscellaneous
- Acute appendicitis
- Inflammatory bowel disease
- Diverticulitis
- UTI
- Mesenteric adenitis
- Nephrolithiasis
- Sexual abuse
- Trauma

History and physical examination
An enquiry into the details of the pain, duration, site of origin, character, severity, aggravating and relieving factors, and radiation should be made. Relationship with the periods and the menstrual cycle should be established. Associated symptoms may include vaginal bleeding, gastrointestinal symptoms (nausea, vomiting, constipation, dyschezia, and anorexia), fever, back pain, or urinary symptoms (frequency, urgency, and dysuria). A past history of PID, infertility, and pelvic surgery may be relevant. The history is a good guide to the likely cause and helps to plan the investigations.

Acute pelvic pain tends to present as a medical emergency. The degree of urgency depends on the severity of the pain and the patient's vital signs. Unstable patients or those in severe pain should be suspected of having a ruptured tubal pregnancy (if pregnancy test is positive), tubo-ovarian cyst/mass/abscess, or a haemorrhagic ovarian cyst. The vital signs, however, tend to be normal unless the patient has had significant bleeding or is in septic shock.

General examination includes assessment of the patient's pulse, blood pressure, and temperature. Pyrexial patients should be suspected of having an infectious cause, such as PID, pyelonephritis, appendicitis, or diverticulitis. Abdominal palpation may reveal tenderness or a palpable mass. There may be guarding, rebound, or rigidity suggestive of localised or generalised peritonitis. Loin palpation may reveal tenderness in patients with urolithiasis or pyelonephritis.

Examination of the external genitalia tends to be normal, though there may be evidence of bleeding. Internal pelvic examination may yield clues to diagnosis. Cervical motion tenderness may be found in PID, ectopic pregnancy, or adnexal masses, as well as in endometriosis. The uterus may be enlarged in patients with fibroids, adenomyosis, or in pregnant women. Adnexal palpation may reveal tenderness or a mass.

A speculum examination is also useful. A purulent discharge is suggestive of PID. Bleeding on the other hand may suggest a miscarriage or a tubal pregnancy. On occasion the cervix may be dilated with the products of conception protruding through the cervical os as in spontaneous miscarriage.

Investigations and management
- *Urine pregnancy test.* Helps differentiate pregnancy-related causes from gynaecological and miscellaneous causes of acute pelvic pain.
- *FBC.* Neutrophilia is a useful clue to suspect underlying infections. Anaemia resulting from a ruptured ectopic or a haemorrhagic ovarian cyst may also be detected.
- *Urine microscopy and culture.* Provides clues to an underlying urological cause for the pain.
- *USS of the pelvis.* Is useful for detecting early pregnancy-related problems, adnexal masses, and uterine fibroids as an underlying cause of the pain.

The investigation and diagnosis of ectopic pregnancy, a life threatening cause for acute pelvic pain, has been dealt with in greater detail in the chapter 'Problems in Early Pregnancy'. Management of patients depends on the severity and duration of pain. Mild pain may require simple analgesia over a short period. An underlying infective process such as PID, UTI, appendicitis, or diverticulitis requires antibiotics.

Referral to secondary care
- Where a diagnosis cannot be established
- When surgical intervention is likely to be required
- Patient is haemodynamically unstable
- No response to management in primary care
- Differentiating between a gynaecological cause and appendicitis is an important consideration when making a referral

Management in secondary care
- In acute PID when a patient is vomiting or is not responding to oral antibiotics, intravenous antibiotics are commenced along with supportive treatment.
- Laparoscopy has both a diagnostic and therapeutic role in severe cases of pelvic pain where there is uncertainty about the diagnosis. Ectopic pregnancies, haemorrhagic ovarian cysts, and adnexal masses may be dealt with at laparoscopy.
- When surgical procedures are not possible laparoscopically or are technically difficult, a laparotomy may be needed.

Useful tips
Investigations
○ Urine pregnancy test – to exclude ectopic pregnancy
○ FBC – infections, anaemia
○ Mid-stream urine for microscopy and culture and sensitivity – UTI
○ USS of the pelvis – pregnancy, adnexal masses, fibroids
○ Laparoscopy

Treatment
- Analgesia ± anti-pyretics
- Antibiotics – PID
- Laparoscopy/laparotomy to deal with the cause

Chronic Pelvic Pain

Chronic pelvic pain is defined as constant or intermittent, cyclic or acyclic pain that persists for six months or more and includes dysmenorrhoea, deep dyspareunia, and intermenstrual pain. It is a common condition with a prevalence of 38/1000 women aged between 15–73.

Few presenting symptoms have such a broad differential diagnosis. CPP requires a detailed knowledge of myriad diseases. Patients with CPP are usually evaluated and treated by gynaecologists, gastroenterologists, surgeons, urologists, and physicians. In many patients with CPP the examination and investigations remain unrevealing and no specific cause of the pain can be identified. A multidisciplinary approach to the management is ideal.

Aetiology
Gynaecological causes
- Endometriosis
- Adenomyosis
- Pelvic congestion
- Leiomyomas
- PID

Gastrointestinal causes
- Irritable bowel syndrome
- Diverticular disease
- Inflammatory bowel disease, including coeliac disease

Urological causes
- Interstitial cystitis
- Urethral syndrome
- Chronic urethritis
- Urolithiasis

Musculoskeletal causes
- Myofascial pain syndromes
- Fibromyalgia
- Low back pain
- Osteoporosis

Neurological causes
- Disc herniation
- Spine neoplasms
- Herpes zoster

History
Because of the wide range of possible diagnoses, a detailed history and physical examination are imperative. As with any form of pain, details of its site of origin, character, severity, aggravating and relieving factors, radiation, and effect on daily living need to be noted.

The location of the pain can be misleading because the visceral innervation of pelvic organs shares common pathways along the sacral plexus and dorsal nerve roots of the thoracolumbar spine. Uterine pain may radiate down the front of the thigh.

Gynaecological disorders
Pain occurring cyclically and in association with the periods indicates a gynaecological cause.
- Abnormal vaginal bleeding (irregular or excessive) or a sudden onset of dysmenorrhoea may indicate an underlying endometriosis, fibroid, or adenomyosis.
- Patients with dyspareunia, a common co-existing complaint in women with CPP, need to be questioned in greater detail. Whereas introital pain, or pain at the time of penetration, is associated with vaginismus and vulvar vestibulitis, deep dyspareunia has a much wider aetiology. Deep dyspareunia may be associated with endometriosis, fixed uterine retroversion, irritable bowel syndrome, adhesions, interstitial cystitis, or urethritis.
- Deep dyspareunia associated with post-coital ache and CPP of a variable nature and location with exacerbations on standing may be suggestive of pelvic congestion syndrome.

Pelvic adhesions
A history of previous abdominal surgery or pelvic infections may suggest pelvic adhesions. Only dense adhesions involving the bowel are believed to be a potential cause of CPP. Patients may have cyclical pain or even bleeding from a surgical scar indicative of endometriosis implants in the scar tissue.

Urological disorders
Symptoms of dysuria, frequency, incontinence, or incomplete emptying necessitate further urological investigation.
- Interstitial cystitis represents a clinical syndrome with symptoms that include urgency, frequency, suprapubic pain, and voiding symptoms can be worse with intercourse.

- The urethral syndrome is associated with urethral tenderness, dysuria, frequency, and incomplete voiding.
- A palpable urethral mass is indicative of urethral diverticulum.
- Patients with urethritis may have sterile pyuria if the organisms are mycoplasma, ureaplasma, or Chlamydia, since these are difficult to grow in cultures.
- Recurrent haematuria around menstruation may be a sign of endometriosis involving the urinary tract.

Gastrointestinal tract disorders
- The pain of irritable bowel syndrome tends to be colicky and associated with a sensation of rectal fullness or incomplete emptying. It follows a relapsing course pattern of bloating and cramping with alterations in stool frequency and/or consistency. It is improved with bowel movements but may be intensified by meals. The pain is often worse around the time of menstruation and may be associated with dyspareunia. These patients may give a history of certain foods worsening or inducing their symptoms. These sensitivities might include a high fat diet, lactose, sorbitol, caffeine, or alcohol excess. They do not represent true food allergies as much as an exaggerated gastric colonic reflex that is brought on by the particular food products. When the small bowel is involved, pain is often located around the periumbilical region or the right lower quadrant. Colon involvement may cause pain in either or both lower quadrants.
- Patients with ulcerative colitis present with cramping that is relieved by voluminous, often bloody diarrhoea. Inflammatory bowel conditions may cause tenderness at the apex of the vagina with resulting dyspareunia.
- The pain of diverticular disease is usually in the left lower quadrant and improves with bowel movement and the passage of flatus.

Neurological and psychiatric disorders
Myofascial pain syndromes are characterised by hypersensitive or tender spots that are referred to as 'trigger points'. Though it tends to present more commonly as chronic low back pain, shoulder pain, or neck pain, it may present as CPP.

The typical symptom of pelvic floor myalgia is that of pelvic discomfort often described as a pressure. The patient reports problems with urinary hesitancy, and history of the discomfort being made worse with prolonged sitting, particularly on hard surfaces. Another key symptom is dyspareunia with post-coital ache. On examination these patients have difficulty in demonstrating a simple squeeze or relaxation. In addition, the muscles are quite tender to palpation. Fibromyalgia presents as a more diffuse pelvic pain.

CPP is a somatoform disorder, hence the psychiatric and social history is of vital importance. Women with history of childhood or lifetime sexual abuse have a higher incidence of CPP. A past history of abuse or victimisation may be obtained with sensitivity and patience. The presence of multiple symptoms may suggest a primarily psychiatric diagnosis.

Useful tips

Clue to diagnosis	Possible diagnosis
Cyclic pain associated with periods	Gynaecologic origin
Abnormal vaginal bleeding and/or sudden onset dysmenorrhoea	Endometriosis, functional ovarian cyst, adenomyosis, fibroids
Superficial dyspareunia	Vaginismus, vulvar vestibulitis, cyclic vulvovaginitis
Deep dyspareunia	Endometriosis, fixed uterine retroversion, irritable bowel syndrome, pelvic adhesions, interstitial cystitis or urethritis, pelvic congestion syndrome
Crampy abdominal pain with bloatedness alternating with diarrhoea and constipation	Irritable bowel syndrome
Melaena, rectal bleeding	Inflammatory bowel disease
Previous surgery/pelvic infections	Pelvic adhesions
Cyclical pain and/or bleeding from a surgical scar	Scar endometriosis
Urethral tenderness/dysuria	Urethral syndrome
Multiple somatic complaints	Sexual abuse, psychiatric disorder

Physical examination

Talking the patient through the examination process helps decrease the anticipatory guarding reflex commonly seen in patients with CPP.

The abdomen is palpated in the usual manner, starting in the zone opposite to the area of maximum pain. The patient is asked to point out the area of maximum pain and an attempt to reproduce this during abdominal palpation is made. Asking the patient to lift her heels off the examination table in the supine position splints the intra-abdominal organs from palpation. If pain is still experienced during this manoeuvre, abdominal wall pathology is more likely. Gently pinching the skin in the dermatomes starting from T10 down to S5 may elicit a hyperaesthetic dermatome, which may respond to trigger point injections. Both the groins should be palpated to rule out enlarged lymph nodes arising either from an infection or neoplasia.

After abdominal examination is complete, a pelvic examination is performed. The vulva is examined externally for redness, trauma, and signs of infection or pelvic relaxation. Asking the patient to bear down while separating the labia makes pelvic relaxation obvious. Following external inspection, a speculum examination with a warm and lubricated speculum is performed. For the narrow introitus, a small sized speculum should be used. Difficulty in inserting the speculum is indicative of vaginismus or deep dyspareunia. Conversely, the lack of difficulty with speculum examination followed by marked difficulty with digital examination is suggestive of a history of physical or sexual abuse.

Vaginismus may be apparent on digital examination. Palpation of the cervix may elicit tenderness. Any pelvic pathology associated with inflammation or fixation of the cervix and/or other structures in the pouch of Douglas may cause tenderness; e.g. endometriosis, pelvic adhesive disease, inflammatory bowel disease. A fixed retroverted uterus can occasionally be a cause for the pain.

After vaginal examination, a bimanual palpation of the uterus indicates the size, mobility, and position of the uterus. An enlarged, tender uterus is seen classically in adenomyosis. A fibroid uterus, though enlarged, is rarely tender unless undergoing degenerative changes.

Palpation of the uterosacral ligaments at rectovaginal examination may reveal areas of nodularity or thickening, strongly suggestive of endometriosis.

Useful tips

Clue to diagnosis	Possible diagnosis
Abdominal wall tenderness that persists on splinting	Abdominal wall pathology
Hypersensitive area noted on skin pinching	Trigger point pain
Lateral vaginal wall tenderness	Pelvic floor tension myalgia
Pain on speculum examination	Vaginismus, other causes of dyspareunia
Adnexal masses and/or tenderness	Endometriosis, pelvic adhesive disease, chronic PID/tubo-ovarian masses, rarely pelvic kidney
Fixed retroverted uterus	Endometriosis, PID, previous surgery
Enlarged uterus	Fibroid, adenomyosis
Nodularity of uterosacral ligaments	Endometriosis
Palpable urethral mass	Urethral diverticulum
Low backache	Musculoskeletal pain
Suprapubic tenderness	Interstitial cystitis

Investigations

Primary care

Investigations are tailored to the patient depending on the history and physical examination. Maintaining a pain diary for one to two months is useful in establishing the cyclical nature of the CPP.

FBC allows a determination of infectious and inflammatory processes. And for patients in whom pelvic examination has been unsatisfactory either due to obesity or patient-related anxiety, a pelvic USS may yield some useful information. It may identify leiomyomas or adenomyomas as a possible cause for pelvic pain. It is also useful in the detection of adnexal cysts or mass. Often a negative USS is enough to reassure the patient.

Genital swabs should be taken to screen for gonorrhoea, Chlamydia, and bacterial vaginosis. Urinalysis and culture and sensitivity should also be performed in women with history suggestive of urological cause.

Secondary care
Laparoscopy is useful in diagnosing pelvic pathology. It is important to understand its limitations, however. In approximately 39% of women the laparoscopy can be negative. In addition, the lesions are heterogeneous and therefore the accuracy of diagnosis is dependent on the abilities of the surgeon. Many women will be reassured by a negative laparoscopy and their pain will subside without any treatment.

Cystourethroscopy may be indicated where symptoms appear to be of a urological nature even though no diagnosis was reached following initial workup.

Barium enema is diagnostic in patients suspected to have inflammatory bowel disease. It is also useful in the diagnosis of diverticular disease. Irritable bowel syndrome is a diagnosis of exclusion and there are no specific laboratory tests to make a diagnosis.

Useful tips
- Laboratory tests: FBC, C reactive protein, triple swabs, MSU
- USS: leiomyomas, adenomyomas, adnexal cysts, ovarian masses
- Laparoscopy: endometriosis, pelvic congestion syndrome, pelvic adhesive disease
- Barium enema: inflammatory bowel disease, diverticular disease

---

Treatment
Primary care
Simple analgesia is the first step in women with no apparent cause on primary investigations. In women with no contraindications to the Pill, the COCP can be tried as a first-line treatment. Putting women in touch with self-help groups and information leaflets is helpful, too.

In all patients with suspected endometriosis, medical treatment should be considered prior to referral. The medical treatment of endometriosis is directed towards simple analgesia or suppression of ovulation. The RCOG recommends using NSAIDs (e.g. mefenamic acid) as a first-line approach because often this may be all that is needed for patients with mild endometriosis. Patients desirous of contraception may be prescribed the COCP (assuming there are no contraindications), given back to back without withdrawal bleeding. This should be given initially for six months.

If all these empiric forms of treatment fail, referral to a gynaecologist should be considered. In patients with associated fertility concerns however, referral should be earlier rather than later. Failing these initial forms of medical treatment, a trial of GnRH analogues may be considered for three to six months in primary care.

The treatment of irritable bowel syndrome is symptomatic. In patients with crampy pain, anti-spasmodics such as dicyclomine or hyoscine are beneficial. The anti-spasmodic mebeverine (135mg tds orally) is also widely used for the treatment of irritable bowel syndrome. Patients complaining primarily of gaseous distension and cramping may benefit from simethicone or peppermint oil. If the predominant symptom is diarrhoea however, fibre supplements are very beneficial. For constipation, a bulking laxative is useful. Adequate fluid intake should be emphasised. Stress is an important factor that can bring on symptoms in those that suffer with irritable bowel syndrome. Hence changes in lifestyle habits and psychological therapy can bring about a favourable change in the condition. Some SSRIs have been shown to be effective in treating irritable bowel syndrome; other, newer serotonin modulating agents are currently under evaluation.

Secondary care
There is evidence that counselling supported by ultrasound scanning is associated with reduced pain and improvement in mood. In most cases, the diagnosis is established by laparoscopy. In one-third of women, endometriosis is diagnosed, and the treatment depends on the desire for fertility, severity of the disease, age of the patient, etc.

Medical treatment options include progestogens, COCP (back-to-back), GnRH analogues with or without add back hormone replacement for 6–12 months, and analgesics. Surgical options include excision/ablation of endometriosis, cystectomy of endometriomas, or oophorectomy. The radical treatment consists of pelvic clearance that involves total abdominal hysterectomy and bilateral salpingo-oophorectomy.

Adhesiolysis does not provide symptom relief other than where the adhesions are dense. PID might cause tubo-ovarian mass, which requires salpingo-oophorectomy or a pelvic clearance if the symptoms are severe, the disease is bilateral, or there are dense adhesions. Women suspected to have pelvic congestion syndrome can have a trial with medroxyprogesterone acetate 30–50mg daily over a three-to-six-month period. Because the condition is believed to be a stress-related ovarian-dependent functional disturbance, stress management and psychotherapy have also been shown to be beneficial.

For patients with ovarian/internal iliac varices, transcatheter embolotherapy provides a new non-surgical treatment option. There is a significant decrease in pain based on visual analogue scale without any notable impact on the menstrual cycle.

When there is no visible pelvic pathology, neuroablative procedures like LUNA and presacral neurectomy are offered by gynaecologists. Though presacral neurectomy provides better pain relief, it is associated with a high risk of complications. The evidence for effectiveness of LUNA is not strong and results from current randomised trials are awaited. In women who undergo hysterectomy for CPP without visible pathology, up to 15% have persistent pelvic pain post-operatively.

Treatment of pelvic floor tension myalgia includes traditional therapies; i.e. localised heat, muscle relaxants, and neurolytic therapy. Amitriptyline or other tricyclics are particularly beneficial. Trigger point therapy is important in the management of myofascial pain syndromes. If conservative therapy is unable to eradicate the pain, an injection of 0.5% lignocaine, using a series of three to five injections is extremely beneficial and also diagnostic.

However, in the absence of positive results a referral must be considered to the appropriate specialists. Patients with CPP, which is resistant to usual management, are referred to the pain clinics that are staffed by anaesthetists, pain nurses, pain psychologist, and occasionally an interested gynaecologist. In women with dyspareunia and underlying history of sexual abuse, consultation with a psychosexual counsellor is helpful.

Useful tips
Algorithm for management of CPP

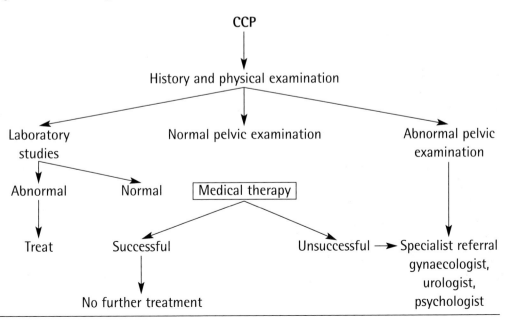

Medical treatments

○ Endometriosis: NSAIDs, COCP, depot medroxyprogesterone acetate, GnRH analogues
○ Uterine retroversion: trial of Smith–Hodge pessary
○ Cyclic vulvovaginitis: fluconazole 150mg weekly for 3–6 months
○ Vulvar vestibulitis: topical steroids
○ Dysesthetic vulvodynia: neurolytic agents (amitriptyline)
○ Pelvic floor tension myalgia: localised heat, muscle relaxants, neurolytic therapy
○ Vaginismus: graduated vaginal dilators
○ Recurrent ovarian cysts: COCP
○ Pelvic trigger points: local injection of 0.5% lignocaine 3–5 injections
○ Bile salt-related colitis following cholecystotomy: cholestyramine
○ Irritable bowel syndrome with severe cramping: anti–spasmodics
○ Irritable bowel syndrome with irregular bowels: fibre supplements
○ Pelvic congestion syndrome: medroxyprogesterone 30–50mg daily for 3–6 months

Further Reading

1. Zondervan KT, Yudkin PL, Vessey MP, *et al.* The community prevalence of chronic pelvic pain in women and associated illness behaviour. *BJGP* 2001; **51(468):** 541-547.
2. Luzzi G, O'Leary M. Chronic pelvic pain syndrome. *BMJ* 1999; **318:** 1227-1228.
3. Stones RW, Mountfield J. Interventions for treating chronic pelvic pain in women (Cochrane Review). In: *The Cochrane Library,* Issue 4. Oxford: Update Software, 2002.
4. Longstreth GF, Drossman DA. New developments in the diagnosis and treatment of irritable bowel syndrome. *Curr Gastroenterol Rep* 2002; **4(5):** 427-434.
5. Howard FM. The role of laparoscopy in CPP: promise and pitfalls. *Obstet Gynecol Surv* 1993; **48:** 357-387.
6. Steege JF, Stout AL, Somkuti SG. CPP in women: towards an integrative model. *Obstet Gynecol Surv* 1993; **48:** 95-110.
7. Gambone JC, Mittman BS, Munro MG, *et al.* Consensus statement for the management of chronic pelvic pain and endometriosis: proceedings of an expert-panel consensus process. *Fertil Steril* 2002; **78(5):** 961-972.

Useful Websites

• Women's Health provides health information on a variety of gynaecological health issues, some of which are related to pelvic pain. Women's Health is a national voluntary organisation. They provide a helpline and enquiry service, newsletter, a series of health information leaflets, a reference library, and a self-help support network. URL: http://www.womenshealthlondon.org.uk/links.html.
• The International Pelvic Pain Society provides information for physicians and also a downloadable patient information booklet on CPP. URL: http://www.pelvicpain.org/.

Subfertility

Dr Pallavi M Latthe and Mr Stephen Keay

Introduction

Subfertility is defined as the inability to conceive after one year of unprotected sexual intercourse. Approximately one-in-six couples in the UK will experience involuntary subfertility at some stage during their lives.

The highest chance of conceiving is in a couple's first month of unprotected intercourse (33%); thereafter the monthly fecundity is 25%. Overall, 90% of couples will have conceived after one year, rising to 95% after two years.

Practitioners would investigate a couple after 12 months, but earlier investigations and referral are justified in women aged 35 years or above and/or if there are significant risk factors identified in their history or abnormalities detected on clinical examination.

The causes of infertility and their approximate frequency.

Cause	Frequency (%)[a]
Sperm defects or dysfunction	30
Ovulation failure (amenorrhoea or oligomenorrhoea)	25
Tubal infective damage	20
Unexplained infertility	25
Endometriosis (causing structural pelvic damage)	5
Coital failure or infrequency	5
Cervical mucus defects or dysfunction	3
Uterine abnormalities (such as fibroids or abnormalities of shape)	<1

[a]Total exceeds 100% as 15% of couples have more than one cause of subfertility.

Adapted from Hull M *et al*. Population study of causes, treatment, and outcome of infertility. *BMJ* 1985; **291**: 1693–1697, with permission from the BMJ Publishing Group.

Factors Adversely Affecting Fertiltity
- Advanced female age
- Smoking
- Duration of subfertility

General practitioners are usually the first of the medical professionals to see a couple who have concerns about their fertility. Ideally, both partners should attend the initial consultation and have their history and examination carried out. This may be impracticable if the couple are registered with different practices, but it should be emphasised they both require investigations. As well, it should be established that the couple has regular intercourse (2–3 per week) and that they understand when in the menstrual cycle they are most likely to conceive.

Increasingly, local protocols are being developed between primary and secondary care based on national guidelines, to ensure appropriate investigations are conducted at the correct time and to eliminate duplication of tests. Local guidelines, if available, may help practitioners in their initial management of the couple and ensure consistency in investigation.

Though the initial consultation provides an opportunity for general pre-pregnancy advice, clinical history and examination frequently give no indication of the cause of the couple's subfertility and the aetiology may only be apparent after the results of investigations are available. An abnormal finding in either partner is sufficient to refer to a dedicated specialist infertility clinic.

Key Points in History
Female
- Previous pregnancies and outcome
- Previous PID or infective complications of pregnancy – tubal infective damage
- Previous contraception and any problems (such as 'lost' IUCD)
- Surgical history (such as ovarian cyst, appendicectomy)
- Dysmenhorrhoea +/- deep dyspareunia - endometriosis
- Infrequent or absent periods – anovulation
- Current medical illness
- Drug treatments – prescribed and 'recreational'
- Diet
- Smoking, alcohol consumption, excessive caffeine intake
- Galactorrhoea
- Coital frequency and timing

Male
- Occupation (exposure to excessive heat or toxin, such as cellulose thinners)
- Medical history (such as mumps, venereal infections)

- Current medical illness
- Erectile or ejaculatory difficulty
- Groin or testicular surgery or delay in descent of testes – sperm dysfunction
- Prescribed drug treatments (such as sulfasalazine)
- Lifestyle habits – drug misuse (such as anabolic steroids), smoking, alcohol consumption, excessive caffeine intake

Childhood cancer

- Survivors of childhood cancer have a long-term risk of subfertility and should have early referral for infertility investigation and treatment. Female survivors are at increased risk of premature menopause, while male survivors will have reduced spermatogenesis.

Initial investigations in primary care.

Who	Test	When and why
Male (all)	Seminal fluid analysis	After 3 days' abstinence; a second sample 4-6 weeks later is recommended to rule out or confirm male factor subfertility
Female (all)	Vaginal and endocervical swabs	Any stage; treat if positive and refer
	Progesterone	Mid-luteal phase (7 days prior to the next expected period) to assess for ovulation
	Rubella immunity	As soon as possible; give rubella vaccine if non-immune with contraception for a month
	FBC	Any stage; treat if anaemic
Female (oligo or amenorrhoea)	FSH	Day 2, 3, or 4 of menstrual cycle (random if amenorrhoea); assess ovarian reserve; if raised indicates (incipient) ovarian failure
	LH, testosterone	Day 2, 3, or 4 of menstrual cycle; if raised (with normal FSH) suggests PCOS
	Prolactin	Checks for hyperprolactinaemia; if marginally raised with regular cycles may suggest PCOS; if raised with amenorrhoea suggests prolactinoma; referral to reproductive endocrinologist if drug-induced cause excluded

The majority of women who give history of regular periods between 23 and 35 days are likely to be ovulating. The observation of a thinning in cervical mucus is one of the best indirect indicators of ovulation and can be useful in pinpointing the most fertile time. When there is history of oligomenorrhoea, anovulation is likely and serum progesterone is of limited value, as predicting the mid-luteal phase is difficult. Oligomenorrhoeic women should have basal FSH, LH, testosterone, and prolactin measured; also thyroid function tests should be checked. PCOS is associated with high basal LH concentrations (>10IU/l) and high androstenedione; high basal FSH levels (>30IU/l) indicates ovarian failure, which is a rare but important cause of amenorrhoea. In normal healthy women without infertility problems, a FSH level up to 10 would be considered normal – a healthy normal would be 5–6 – but the normal varies with age such that a level of 8 in a 35-year-old would be reasonable but would be considered abnormal in a 20-year-old.

Thyroid function tests and prolactin should NOT be checked routinely in women with regular menstrual cycles.

Midluteal progesterone concentrations should be interpreted after the next period confirming that the sample was correctly timed. Levels >30nmol/l can be considered ovulatory. If the level is between 16–30nmol/l the blood test should be repeated in a further cycle, with a second measurement, if necessary, two days after the first. Progesterone levels consistently <30nmol/l are indication to refer to an infertility clinic for controlled ovarian stimulation.

Chlamydia serology can be performed to screen for potential tubal infective damage (N-<1:128) in women with past history of chlamydial infection or multiple sexual partners; if raised, treat both partners with antibiotics and refer early to the specialist.

The male partner should have two semen analyses four weeks apart performed in a dedicated andrology laboratory, preferably associated with the hospital to which the GP refers their patients. Some medications will reduce sperm counts; e.g. H_2 antagonists and spironolactone.

Seminal fluid analysis.

Parameter	Normal	If abnormal
Volume	2–5 ml	If low – incomplete collection
Count	>20 x 106	Repeat; check no acute/chronic illness; advice on smoking, alcohol, loose underwear; refer if repeat abnormal
Motility	>50% progressive	Repeat; check that sample was not collected in condom or unconventional container; refer early
Morphology	>15% normal forms	Repeat and refer

The post-coital test is not recommended and urinary LH kits are expensive and are of no proven benefit in improving conception rates.

Pre-Pregnancy Advice
- *Smoking.* Women should be advised and supported to give up.
- *Folic acid.* Supplements (400mcg daily) should be taken by women to reduce the risk of foetal neural tube defects. A higher dose of 5mg daily is advised if the patient has had a previous child with a neural tube defect.
- *Rubella.* Immunity should be tested – if low or non-immune, vaccination should be offered and conception avoided for one month after vaccination.
- *Alcohol.* Intake should be no more than two units per week for women and men should not drink to excess either.
- *Recreational drugs.* Can reduce fertility; e.g. cannabis can affect sperm motility.
- *Weight.* Women with a body mass index >30 should attempt to lose weight whether they have a regular menstrual cycle or not. In anovulatory women with PCOS, a modest reduction in weight through a programme of calorie restriction and regular exercise may help in restoring spontaneous ovulation or permit easier induction of ovulation with clomiphene. Obesity has implications for pregnancy and delivery too, should treatment be successful.

Treatment in Primary Care
- It is acceptable to defer referral if the woman is <35 years old and the couple's history, examination, and initial investigations are all normal and their duration of infertility is <18 months' duration.
- For anovulation, the first-line treatment of infrequent ovulation is with the anti-oestrogen clomiphene citrate. It acts mainly by blocking oestrogen receptors in the pituitary, which promotes the release of additional FSH and consequently follicular development. Clomiphene 50mg is administered from day 2–6 of the menstrual cycle and ideally the response should be assessed by ultrasound. With the DoH's recommendation of a maximum of six cycles of clomiphene use, it is more appropriate that this is carried out under supervision of a specialist infertility clinic rather than in primary care.
- The support and counselling required during investigation and treatment should not be underestimated and a plan for continued support in primary care after referral is helpful.

Indications for early referral to specialist fertility clinic
- *Age.* Female partners 35 years or over.
- *Duration.* Subfertility for three years or more.
- *History.* Any significant factors in the past history in either partner, especially if the female's periods are absent or irregular or she has a history of pelvic infection or previous abdominal surgery.

- *Investigations.* Abnormal seminal fluid analysis, raised FSH or/and LH (>10IU/l) in early follicular phase, chlamydia antibody titre >1:256.

In the referral letter to the secondary or tertiary infertility centre, the GP should include the results of initial screening tests (it is important to state the actual results, e.g. FSH level, rather than just stating that they are normal) and mention the past obstetric, medical, and surgical as well as personal history of the female along with details of pregnancies fathered by the male partner. The GP should also mention concerns about the suitability of the couple for further treatment with details on past history of sexual or physical abuse. The HFEA requires a statement on potential problems that might affect the 'welfare of the unborn child' before any assisted conception treatment is provided.

Investigations in Secondary Care
Female
- Endocrine profile by the GP is not repeated unless abnormal. An elevated prolactin is repeated to ensure that it was not due to stress and if over 1000mIU/l then MRI of the pituitary fossa is performed along with examination of the visual fields.
- FSH >10IU/l implies a reduced ovarian reserve is likely and is associated with poorer outcomes at IVF.
- A transvaginal scan may be performed to assess the ovaries for cysts and to look for typical polycystic ovaries.
- Tubal patency is usually assessed by laparoscopy and dye test but hysterosalpingography or hysterocontrastsonography can be used as an alternative.
- If uterine anomaly or presence of fibroids is suspected, a hysteroscopy can be carried out.
- Prior to uterine instrumentation, women are screened for infection with vaginal and endocervical swab (for Chlamydia), if this has not already been done in primary care. Antibiotic prophylaxis is given to screen positive women.

Male
- If the two SFA results are normal, then no further tests are performed.
- If SFA is abnormal, clinical examination is then carried out for secondary sexual characteristics, testicular size, varicocele, and absent or abnormal vas. Karyotype and cystic fibrosis screen is performed for those with azoospermia or severe oligospermia (<5 x 10^6/ml).
- In case of oligoasthenoteratozoospermia or azoospermia, full hormonal profile including FSH, testosterone, and prolactin is performed.
- If the ejaculate shows recurrent infection, it is sent for microbiological assessment and the man with his partner is referred to a GUM clinic for further screening and treatment.
- If testicular examination is abnormal, a urological opinion should be sought +/- a scrotal ultrasound performed.

- There remains a 20% chance of spontaneous conception even in the presence of sperm dysfunction and this should be considered when discussing the effectiveness of any intervention.

Treatment in Secondary and Tertiary Care

Anovulation

If anovulation is the sole abnormality, ovulation is induced with an anti-oestrogen. Clomiphene is the usual first-line treatment, although tamoxifen can occasionally be used as an alternative. Clomiphene 50mg daily from days 2–6 inclusive is prescribed and the response monitored by transvaginal ultrasound and serum progesterone (sampled seven days following presumed ovulation). The dose can be increased to 100mg or 150mg if no response occurs, but at higher doses there may be an adverse effect upon cervical mucus receptivity. Up to 80% of women will ovulate on clomiphene – up to 10% of conceptions will be multiple.

If clomiphene fails to induce ovulation the options are to use gonadotrophins or adopt a surgical approach with ovarian diathermy. The surgical approach is intended to induce spontaneous mono-ovulation and consequently a low multiple pregnancy rate. There are a variety of gonadotrophin stimulation regimes, but often the threshold between no response and an over-response is very narrow. Ultrasound monitoring is mandatory and cancellation of cycles in which multiple follicles develop is crucial in preventing multiple pregnancy.

Metformin is an insulin-sensitising agent that has been used in overweight women with PCOS and has restored menstruation and ovulation. It has also proven worthwhile in women with high insulin resistance. The exact indications for and success of metformin will only be clear once the results of RCTs are available.

In women with premature menopause or high FSH levels (poor ovarian reserve) oocyte donation by a close relative or unknown donor is a viable option.

Tubal infertility

The success rates for reconstructive tubal surgery are poor (15–20%) and careful patient selection is important. Infective tubal damage with hydrosalpinges is a particularly unrewarding group. IVF offers a more effective treatment in most cases, although proximal tubal occlusion may be amenable selective salpingography and transcervical tubal cannulation.

Sperm dysfunction

Intrauterine insemination combined with superovulation may be carried out for 'borderline male subfertility', but for significant sperm dysfunction the most effective treatment is ICSI.

Azoospermic men may undergo PESA or TESA to retrieve sperm prior to ICSI. The follow-up of children born by this method of treatment is ongoing, as an excess of sex chromosome abnormalities has been detected.

The success of ICSI has lead to a reduction in the demand for intrauterine insemination with donor sperm, but this remains a viable alternative if no sperm are retrieved surgically or genetic abnormalities are present in the male.

Endometriosis
Medical treatment of minor endometriosis does not improve fertility. Surgical treatment of severe endometriosis to restore the pelvic anatomy can be undertaken laparoscopically or at laparotomy. Alternatively, IVF may be offered. Endometriotic cyst of the ovary >4cm diameter requires surgical treatment.

Unexplained Infertility
This definition applies to those couples in whom no cause is identified after full investigation of both partners. The chance of conceiving spontaneously after three years of trying declines significantly. Both IVF and IUI combined with superovulation are treatment options. IVF provides useful information about fertilisation.

Counselling regarding adoption or remaining childless is very important when treatment has been unsuccessful and should be readily available for couples within a tertiary centre.

Summary points
○ The major causes of subfertility are anovulation, tubal damage, and sperm dysfunction.
○ For most couples, history and examination will be unremarkable and investigations are relied on for indicating cause of the subfertility.
○ GPs have the opportunity to impart preconception advice about smoking, obesity, and folic acid.
○ Women >35 years should be referred early
○ Couples with sperm dysfunction or likely tubal damage should be referred early to secondary or tertiary clinics.

Polycystic Ovarian Syndrome
Around one-in-five women have polycystic ovaries, the term used to describe the appearances of the ovaries when they are seen on USS. PCOS is a condition in which women have polycystic ovaries and symptoms related to it and is the commonest endocrinological condition in women.

The definition of PCOS is controversial. The polycystic ovary is diagnosed on transvaginal ultrasound. The most consistent feature is the peripheral ring of small follicles 2–8mm in diameter with increased ovarian stroma. There is a familial link in PCOS, although the mode of inheritance is not known. Women with PCOS often develop symptoms following weight gain. The polygenic background with involvement of both genetic and environmental factors is expected to play a role in development of PCOS.

Symptoms of polycystic ovarian syndrome
- *Menstrual irregularities.* Anovulation can cause amenorrhoea, oligomenorrhoea, and heavy periods.
- *Subfertility.* Anovulation may occur in women with irregular or absent cycles.
- *Miscarriage.* High levels of circulating LH are implicated in the higher risk of miscarriage in PCOS.
- *Hirsutism.* Due to increased levels of serum androgens, around half the women complain of acne on the face and back, or unwanted hair on the face, chest, arms, and legs.
- *Obesity.*

Features associated with polycystic ovaries
- Acne
- Subfertility
- Hirsutism
- Obesity
- Amenorrhoea
- Increased risk of miscarriage
- Increased risk of diabetes, endometrial hyperplasia, and carcinoma and possibly cardiovascular disease

Investigations
- Serum LH, FSH, prolactin, androstenedione, and testosterone levels during the first four days of menstrual bleeding
- Characteristic appearance of ovaries on ultrasound

Androgen excess
- Testosterone, DHEAS to rule out rare ovarian or adrenal tumours
- 17 alpha hydroxy progesterone to rule out late onset congenital adrenal hyperplasia
- Ultrasound

Investigations of PCOS may show:
- High serum LH with a normal FSH
- Increased serum androgens

○ High free androgen index (i.e. low SHBG)
○ High insulin levels (not measured outside a research setting)
○ High prolactin
○ Characteristic ovarian appearance on ultrasound

Management

All women with polycystic ovaries should try to maintain normal weight. There are also clear benefits of regular aerobic exercise; this is especially true for women who wish to become pregnant, as it can restore ovulation if oligomenorrhoeic. A woman should have a minimum of 3–4 periods a year, whether spontaneous or induced, to reduce the risk of endometrial hyperplasia.

Symptomatic treatment

Menstrual irregularities

For most women with PCOS, COCP forms the backbone of management. If this is unsuitable, cyclical progesterone therapy (D5-25) will help in reducing blood loss in heavy irregular periods. Mirena IUS can be fitted for endometrial protection in women with oligomenorrhoea or heavy irregular periods and also provides contraception.

Benefits of oral contraceptive pill in PCOS
○ Androgen levels reduced
○ SHBG increased
○ Acne and hirsutism reduced
○ Regular withdrawal bleeding
○ Protective effect on endometrium
○ Effective contraception

Subfertility

This relates to oligomenorrhoea. Weight loss if obese is helpful. The investigation and management of anovulation has been discussed previously.

Hirsutism

Ninety per cent of women complaining of hirsutism have polycystic ovaries. Clinical assessment should include the history of onset and speed of progression of hirsutism, menstrual pattern, and drug history. Examination should determine the severity of hirsutism (Ferriman–Gallwey score) and whether there are features of virilisation (breast atrophy, clitoral enlargement, and voice changes). If present, then androgen-secreting tumours should be considered. *Acanthosis nigricans* (pigmented velvety patches in the skin flexures and neck) suggest PCOS with insulin resistance.

Treatment includes advice on weight loss and cosmetic measures like waxing, bleaching, and electrolysis. Women with hirsutism can suffer from low self-esteem and might need psychological support.

Medical treatments may take up to nine months to show improvement – women should be advised of this prior to starting treatment.

The anti-androgen cyproterone acetate has been used with in a low dose of 2mg daily as the progestogenic part of the contraceptive preparation Dianette. Further to this anti-androgen effect, the ethinyl oestradiol component increases SHBG levels, effectively reducing the free androgen. In more severe cases, cyproterone acetate 25–50mg daily can be added to the first days of every cycle packet of Dianette in a reverse sequential scheme. It is important the woman does not conceive while taking cyproterone because of potential effects on a male offspring. Flutamide, spironolactone, and finestaride are infrequently used in the management of hirsutism due to side-effects.

Obesity
It is likely that weight gain in women with PCOS may trigger symptoms and meticulous attention to calorie intake and exercise can lead to weight loss and improvement in symptoms. Orlistat has been used as part of weight reduction programmes in some women with PCOS but is best reserved for women in whom diet and exercise have failed to reduce weight.

Wider health issues
Diabetes mellitus
Hyperinsulinaemia and insulin resistance is implicated in the development of many of the features of PCOS. There is an increased risk of gestational diabetes developing during pregnancy and of NIDDM in late adult life. There may also be a higher risk of developing cardiovascular disease.

Endometrial hyperplasia and cancer
Oestrogenisation in the absence of ovulation (and therefore progesterone) may develop into adenomatous hyperplasia and, ultimately, neoplasia.

Osteoporosis
Women with PCOS are NOT oestrogen deficient and should not be regarded as at risk of osteoporosis.

Ovarian neoplasia
There is some evidence to associate increased risk of borderline ovarian tumours when women with PCOS undergo prolonged pharmacological treatment for ovulation induction

in subfertility (beyond 12–24 months). This forms the basis for the DoH recommendation to limit clomiphene use to six cycles.

Further Reading

1. Royal College of Obstetricians and Gynaecologists. *The Initial Investigation and Management of the Infertile Couple.* [Evidence-based Clinical Guidelines No 6.] London: RCOG Press, 1998.
2. Hull M, Glazener C, Kelly NJ, *et al.* Population study of causes, treatment, and outcome of infertility. *BMJ* 1985; **291**: 1693-1697.
3. Taylor A. The subfertile couple. *Curr Obstet Gynaecol* 2000; **11**: 115-125.
4. Cahill DJ, Wardle PG. Management of infertility. *BMJ* 2002; **325**: 28-32.
5. World Health Organization. *WHO laboratory manual for the examination of human semen and sperm-cervical mucus interaction.* [4th ed.] Cambridge: Cambridge University Press, 1999.
6. Balen A, Jacobs H. *Infertility in Practice.* Edinburgh: Churchill Livingstone, 1997.
7. Hughes E, Collins J, Vandekerckhove P. Clomiphene citrate for unexplained subfertility in women (Cochrane Review). In: *The Cochrane Library,* Issue 2. Oxford: Update Software, 2002.
8. Farquhar C, Vandekerckhove P, Lilford R. Laparoscopic "drilling" by diathermy or laser for ovulation induction in anovulatory polycystic ovary syndrome (Cochrane Review). In: *The Cochrane Library,* Issue 2. Oxford: Update Software, 2002.
9. Eden JA. The polycystic ovary syndrome. *Aust NZ J Obstet Gynaecol* 1989; **29**: 403-416.
10. Heineman MJ. Introduction to polycystic ovary syndrome. *Gynaecology Forum* 1997; **2(2)**: 3-4.
11. Fox R. Polycystic ovarian disease and insulin resistance: pathophysiology and wider health issues. In: Studd J (ed). *Progress in Obstetrics and Gynaecology.* Edinburgh: Churchill Livingstone, 1997; 341-350.
12. Jacobs HS. Hirsutism. *Curr Obstet Gynaecol* 1991; **1**: 217-220.

Useful Websites

- Centre for Reproductive Medicine. URL: http://www.repromed.co.uk.
- UK National Fertility Association. URL: http://www.issue.co.uk.
- Women's Health Information. URL: http://www.womens-health.co.uk/pcos10.htm.
- Verity. URL: http://www.verity-pcos.org.uk.

Family Planning

Dr Rajvir Thandi and Dr Wendy Milligan

Introduction – The GP's Perspective

The ideal method of contraception does not exist, but the GP is ideally placed to provide access to all the methods currently available. A GP does not have to provide contraceptive services but can claim an annual fee for every female patient to whom they give family planning advice. A higher fee is paid if a GP fits a coil. A new claim must be submitted annually and can be made from one month before to six months after the renewal date.

The recognised qualification for general practice in the UK is the DFFP. The training consists of a theoretical course, followed by practical instruction on an individual basis with a training doctor within general practice or in a community clinic. Extra training and practical experience is required to gain a letter of competence to fit coils or implants or to be recognised as a Family Planning Training Doctor. However, there is currently no requirement for a GP to possess any qualification to provide contraceptive services.

A practice nurse who has received family planning training can undertake the majority of the routine follow-up for patients using contraception. Protocols need to be in place, with ready access to a GP if a problem develops.

The availability of hospital– or community-based family planning clinics will vary from area to area. Sometimes special clinics are provided for young people, and often there will be evening or lunch-time sessions. Patients can normally self-refer, or can be referred by the GP if a method is required that the practice does not provide or if a second opinion is needed.

A full range of contraception can be prescribed on an NHS prescription, the FP10, and there is no prescription charge to the patient.

Failure rates are an important part of the discussion that takes place before a particular method is chosen. We need to advise about rates that apply when a method is used perfectly and also the rates that normally apply in practice (see table overleaf). Patients may not always be aware of the range of contraception available and not every method

Pregnancies per 100 women in the first 12 months of use, if used correctly and consistently (based on WHO data).[a]

Condoms	Male	3	(14)
	Female	5	(21)
	Diaphragm	6	(20)
Combined oral contraception		0.1	(0.2–3)
Progestogen oral contraception		0.5	(1–4)
Injectables	Depo-Provera	0.5	–
Implants	Implanon	0.05	–
IUS	Mirena	0.1	–
IUCD	Copper T 380A	0.6	(0.8)
Sterilisation	Male	0.1	(0.2)
	Female	0.5	–
Natural methods		1–9	(25)
No method		85	–

[a]Figures in brackets give failure rates as used in practice.

will appeal to an individual. The GP's role is to provide information and allow an informed choice to be made.

Condoms

Although some primary care organisations provide condoms to be distributed to patients, they cannot be prescribed on an FP10. (They are readily available at community-based clinics, where instruction in their correct use is also available.) Because barriers also protect against sexually transmitted infection, they may be used in addition to other methods. A female polyurethane condom is also available with a similar protective role.

Male condoms are produced in different sizes and are commonly made of latex, which is damaged if exposed to oils and grease. Allergic reactions can develop to the latex or to the coating spermicide. A latex condom without the spermicide or the more expensive polyurethane male condom may then be needed. Patients should be advised to check for a use-by date and the British Standard Kite Mark on the packaging.

Diaphragms and Cervical Caps

A diaphragm needs to be fitted for an individual woman so that the correct size to position it between the posterior fornix and the symphysis pubis is chosen, thus covering the cervix. They should always be used with a spermicide and left in place for six hours after sexual intercourse. The method is now used infrequently but is free of systemic side-effects, although it may be associated with cystitis-like symptoms, as the rim presses on the bladder neck. Diaphragms vary in size from 50–100mm, and the fit should be checked after childbirth or if the user gains or loses a significant amount of weight.

Cervical caps, which fit tightly over the cervix, are also available but are used even less frequently. A specialist clinic is often the best place for a woman to be taught how to use a cap or diaphragm.

Combined Oral Contraception – The Pill

The Pill works by preventing ovulation, in addition to effecting the endometrium, cervical mucus, and possibly tubal function. The first generation of Pills contained high doses of oestrogen and progestogen and was replaced by second generation Pills containing about 30µg of ethinyloestradiol. The third generation was developed to contain less androgenic progestogens and to be less likely to cause or worsen acne, as well as to give good cycle control. They also caused less adverse effects on carbohydrate and lipid metabolism and it was hoped that this would translate into a reduction in arterial wall disease and hypertension. We have no evidence that this is the case and we now know that third generation Pills containing desogestrel and gestodene are more likely to cause venous thromboembolism. Pills containing the newer progestogens norgestimate and the recently introduced drospirenone were not part of the 1995 study, which highlighted this difference in risk. The table below shows the slight increase in risk, which will always be considerably less than that associated with pregnancy.

Risk of venous thromboembolism per 100,000 women.	
Not using combined oral contraception	5
Second generation Pill users	15
Third generation Pill users	25
Pregnancy	60

Before a woman is prescribed oral contraception for the first time, the prescribing doctor must be sure it is appropriate to do so. Careful instruction in its use is also needed and it would be difficult to compress all this into the typical 7–10-minute appointment. Instruction leaflets can provide a helpful reminder, and the FPA provides a particularly good range.

Essential information before the first prescription
1. Age
2. Smoking status
3. Blood pressure
4. BMI
5. LMP and description of usual menstrual cycle
6. Parity
7. Previous contraception use

8. Past medical history:
   • personal history of thrombosis
   • history of headaches or migraine
9. Medication used
10. Family history:
    • thrombosis
    • breast cancer

Contraindications most commonly encountered
 1. Smoker over 35 years (smoker of any age smoking 40 cigarettes daily)
 2. BMI >39 (relative contraindication if >30)
 3. Blood pressure >140/90
 4. Personal history of arterial or venous thrombosis
 5. Surgery with prolonged immobilisation
 6. Migraine with focal symptoms
 7. Breast feeding
 8. History of myocardial infarction or stroke
 9. Diabetes of long duration or with vascular disease
10. Liver disease
11. Breast cancer
12. Age over 49 years
13. Conditions that predispose to thrombosis; e.g. sickle cell disease, active Crohn's
    disease
14. Porphyria
15. Structural heart disease and cardiomyopathy

The above list is not complete, and in cases of doubt a reference text should be consulted or a referral made to the specialist family planning clinic. Sometimes there are relative contraindications, such as a family history of thrombosis or breast cancer, when it is difficult to know if there is an increased risk to the individual. There is a relative risk of breast cancer in Pill users of 1.24 after one year of use, which declines when the Pill is stopped and returns to normal after ten years. Ideally, this should be discussed with the woman, who thus becomes an informed user. A thrombophilia screen can be carried out but may be falsely reassuring, as not all clotting disorders are currently recognised.

The Pill is started on day 1 of the period and continued for 21 days, taken at the same time each day. A seven-day gap then follows, not long enough to permit ovulation but normally long enough to produce a withdrawal bleed. If this PFI is accidentally lengthened by a pill being missed, there is a risk of ovulation and subsequent pregnancy. If the Pill is taken more than 12 hours late, the seven-day rule should be followed; i.e. condoms should be used until the Pill is taken correctly for seven days. When pills are missed in the last seven pills in the pack, it is safer to omit the PFI. Vomiting within two hours of taking the Pill will reduce the amount absorbed, as will severe diarrhoea. In both cases, the seven-day rule should be followed. A maximum of three Pill packets may be run together, omitting the PFI and its withdrawal bleed if either is undesirable (the term 'tri-cycling' is used to describe this).

Which Pill?
As they are associated with a lesser risk of VTE, second generation Pills containing the progestogens levonorgestrel and norethisterone arguably should be first choice. They are also cheaper than third generation Pills. If a woman has acne or hirsuitism, a less androgenic third generation Pill should be offered, as long as the venous thromboembolic effects are discussed and accepted. If a woman has previously used a brand that suited her, that obviously could be her choice again. Phasic Pills are also available, with varying hormone doses throughout the pack. They are more expensive and cause complications if packs need to be run together. MIMS provides a comprehensive table of all available oral contraceptives. It is regularly updated and makes sense of what initially appears to be a bewildering array of brand names.

Side-effects
Nausea may occur but normally settles with continuing use. Breakthrough bleeding also may occur but often settles if the same brand is continued over three months; if not, it may resolve with an increase in the progestogen content of the Pill or a change to another type of progestogen. Initial breast discomfort often settles with continuing use. Headaches related to Pill use often occur in the PFI and up to three packs could be run together with a beneficial effect. A change in episodes of migraine to a more severe type, or one with focal symptoms, would be a reason to stop. Similarly, any symptoms suggestive of thrombosis should result in the Pill being stopped immediately and an urgent referral to hospital for investigation.

Monitoring
The blood pressure should be checked after three months of Pill use, to search for the rare situation when a significant increase occurs. If there are no problems, the woman can then be reviewed on a six-monthly basis. Women are often concerned that the Pill will cause weight gain, and hopefully routine weighing will reassure them or, if not, detect the development of a problem. Routine cervical screening should be encouraged in those who are aged over 20 years.

Progestogen-only Pill – 'the mini-Pill'
The progestogen-only Pill is taken every day, ideally at exactly the same time, although an error of up to three hours can be allowed. The effects are mainly on the endometrium and cervical mucus and they do not consistently prevent ovulation. They have minimal metabolic outcomes and do not cause hypertension or increase thrombosis risk. They are particularly used by breast-feeding women and others in whom oestrogens are

contraindicated. The few contraindications include undiagnosed vaginal bleeding, liver disease, porphyria, and, of course, pregnancy. Specialist advice should be sought for patients with severe cardiovascular disease, breast cancer, or hydatidiform mole. There is an increased risk that any accidental pregnancy may be ectopic, and a possible increased risk of benign ovarian cysts should also be covered in counselling. All progestogen methods can be associated with irregular bleeding. Careful counselling about this feature is essential and increases acceptance of an altered cycle. If ovulation is inhibited, amenorrhoea will ensue and a careful explanation will normally reassure the woman that the mini-Pill is working very well. However, a pregnancy test should be done if there is a concern about irregular pill taking or an interaction that would reduce the mini-Pill's efficacy. If the mini-Pill is taken more than three hours late, the seven-day rule should be followed. Vomiting and severe diarrhoea should be similarly covered.

Emergency Contraception – Levonelle-2

Two 750µg doses of the progestogen levonorgestrel taken 12 hours apart and started within 72 hours of UPSI will provide post-coital contraception. The method works better with a short coitus-to-treatment interval, as it works at the pre-implantation stage.

A trained nurse can decide if emergency contraception should be offered by taking a history and then referring to the GP for a prescription; e.g. under a patient group directive. An example proforma for nurse issuing of emergency contraception is shown at the end of the chapter (p118). A history of multiple episodes of unprotected sex within a cycle is not a reason to withhold emergency contraception for the one occasion that the woman requests it. It should, however, be fully explained that there will be no inhibiting effect on pregnancy as a result of earlier, or later, UPSI.

Percentage of expected pregnancies prevented.

Time	Percentage
≤24 hours	95%
25–48 hours	85%
49–72 hours	58%

It is good practice to arrange a follow-up appointment to ensure no pregnancy has ensued and to discuss future contraception. Pharmacists can provide emergency contraception without a doctor's prescription by selling it to the patient, and in some areas are able to supply it without charge to the patient.

A copper-bearing IUCD can also be inserted up to five days after UPSI or up to day 19 in a 28-day cycle. The IUCD could be removed after the next period or left in place for future contraception. The GP may need to refer to a more experienced colleague or specialist clinic for this method, which has a very low failure rate. Antibiotic prophylaxis at insertion should be considered, as there will not be time to take swabs and await results.

Injectables – Depo-Provera

Depo-Provera (150mg medroxyprogesterone) is a long-acting progestogen given by intra-muscular injection, usually into the gluteal muscle, in the first five days of the cycle. It is licensed to be used at intervals of up to 12 weeks and five days in the UK, although the American licence is for 13 weeks. It can be given immediately after termination of pregnancy or miscarriage but ideally should be postponed until six weeks after childbirth to avoid prolonged bleeding. Obviously, the woman cannot change her mind once the injection has been given, so careful counselling is required. Like all progestogen methods it is associated with altered menstruation, usually amenorrhoea. Ovulation does not occur. Initial irregular bleeding may occur, which can be settled by adding a pack of the combined Pill or bringing the next injection forward. The method is often used by women who cannot remember to take pills and who may also not be good at keeping appointments. If a follow-up appointment is made after an 11-week interval, a woman who forgets to attend can be contacted.

A protocol to manage the woman who attends late for an injection.

Time since last injection	Up to 91 days	92–94 days	95–96 days
If patient has had UPSI	Not at risk	Give emergency contraception	Fit post-coital IUCD
Give injection?	Yes	Yes	Yes

After 96 days the injection should not be given. A pregnancy test should be performed and repeated after a two-week interval in which the patient undertakes not to have UPSI. If both pregnancy tests are negative, Depo-Provera can be given and condoms advised for seven days.

In some women, Depo-Provera use is associated with significant weight gain, when consideration should be given to stopping the method. There can also be a delay of up to one year before periods and normal fertility return when the method is discontinued.

Concerns have been raised about the development of osteoporosis in the long term for Depo-Provera users who develop amenorrhoea. We currently have conflicting evidence on this issue. The risks and benefits in very young women who may not have attained their maximum bone density need careful consideration, but pregnancy itself will cause a reduction in bone density.

Managing bleeding problems that occur with Depo-Provera
- Within four to eight weeks of last injection consider a pack of combined oral contraception if not contraindicated.
- After eight weeks consider giving next injection.
- Use menstrual calendar to record and evaluate bleeding.
- Consider other causes; e.g. Chlamydia.
- If bleeding persists after second injection and is unacceptable, consider alternative method.

Implants – Implanon
Implanon is a single flexible rod, which is fitted under the skin of the upper arm. The implant is 4cm long by 2mm wide and is normally felt in position rather than seen. It has a three-year life and a very good success rate, with its effects reversing quickly upon removal. As well as affecting the endometrium and cervical mucus, Implanon prevents ovulation. It contains 68mg of etonogestrel, which is slowly released to give constant low blood levels. It should be inserted within the first five days of the menstrual cycle, and has the same potential to produce irregular bleeding as all progestogen methods.

Levonorgestrel-Intrauterine System
Marketed under the trade name Mirena in the UK, this is a T-shaped device inserted into the uterus. The upright limb contains a sleeve of levonorgestrel, which exerts its effects mainly locally. Most women will continue to ovulate, and it is the local effects on the endometrium and cervical mucus that prevent pregnancy.

Mirena should be inserted before day 7 of the menstrual cycle and cannot be used post-coitally. It is licensed for five years of use. Because it reduces menstrual blood loss and often produces amenorrhoea, it is also used as a treatment for menorrhagia. Other women rely on it for the progestogen component of HRT (as yet unlicensed in the UK). Unfortunately, it can initially result in irregular bleeding that may persist for three to six months. Because of the expense of the device, careful discussion of this effect should be carried out before insertion.

The presence of the sleeve of hormone results in the need for a wider insertion tube than that required for a conventional IUCD, which can make it more difficult to fit. Like all coils, it should only be fitted if the doctor has been properly trained and has the opportunity to regularly perform insertions.

Drug Interactions with Hormonal Contraception
The BNF provides a comprehensive guide to drug interactions and should always be consulted. Antibiotics only have a detrimental effect on the oestrogen-containing combined Pill. The effects vary, but as the illness being treated may contribute to Pill failure, a case can be made for always following the seven-day rule; i.e. condom use for

the days the antibiotic is taken and also for seven days after it. The woman is advised to continue the combined Pill without having the PFI. The combined Pill can be safely added to tetracycline when it is used in the long term for acne. However, if the tetracycline is added to a combined Pill, condoms should be used for any intercourse in the first three weeks. Drugs that induce liver enzymes could also have an effect on all progestogen methods. These effects may persist for four to eight weeks after the enzyme inducer is stopped.

Commonly encountered drugs that induce liver enzymes.

Anticonvulsants	barbiturates, phenytoin, primidone, carbamazepine, topiramate, oxcarbazepine
Anti-tuberculosis drugs	rifampicin, rifabutin
Anti-fungals	griseofulvin
Protease inhibitors	ritonavir, nelfinavir
Others	lansoprazole, St John's Wort

Use of hormonal contraception with enzyme inducers.

Method	Treatment
Combined oral contraception	Use 1-2 50mcg pills, decrease PFI to 4 days, run 3 packs together
Progestogen-only pills	Not to be used with enzyme-inducing agents; change method or add a condom
Depo-Provera	Reduce interval between injections to 10 weeks
Implants	Possible effect, suggest condom use
IUS	No evidence of reduced efficacy
Progestogen-only emergency contraception	Double first dose of Levonelle-2

Intrauterine Contraceptive Device – 'The Coil'

Effective use of the coil depends on the skill of the fitter as well as the inherent effectiveness of the coil itself. A doctor fitting coils should do so frequently and use a device with a good success rate. The coil's principal effect is the prevention of fertilisation, with a secondary effect on the endometrium preventing implantation.

Most modern IUCDs are small and T-shaped with fine copper wire wrapped around the upright part and sometimes also wrapped around the side arms. They can be fitted more easily in women who have had vaginal deliveries, but it may be possible to fit a coil in a nulliparous woman if one of the smaller coils or a frameless device is used.

Coil insertion is normally carried out within the first five days of the menstrual cycle but can be carried out at any time if there is no risk of pregnancy. Pre-insertion screening for an STI, particularly Chlamydia, may be appropriate. The coil does not cause PID, but insertion may result in a clinical presentation of a previously asymptomatic infection.

Coil fitting should be carried out in a situation that allows the woman to relax and feel at ease. Use of mefenamic acid 500mg before the insertion will reduce cramps. The woman should be encouraged to check for the IUCD threads herself, and attend for a follow-up vaginal examination at 6–12 weeks. If the woman is happy with the method, an annual appointment should then be offered to check the coil remains correctly in place. Coils can be left in place for five to eight years depending on type; however, if they are fitted in a woman over the age of 40 the coil can be left in place until the menopause.

IUCD use is often associated with longer, heavier periods. The coil offers a lesser degree of protection against ectopic pregnancy and a pregnancy test should be carried out if there is irregular bleeding or low abdominal pain.

The coil may be spontaneously expelled unnoticed by the wearer. The absence of threads will alert the wearer that this has happened, although the threads may merely have been drawn up into the cervical canal. The presence of the coil should be located by ultrasound scan and the wearer advised to use condoms until the coil is confirmed to be within the uterus.

The IUCD is removed easily by gentle traction on the threads and its contraceptive effects reverse quickly. It is preferable to remove it during a period. If a pregnancy occurs with the coil in-situ, it should be removed if possible, as this will reduce the risk of second trimester pregnancy loss and premature labour. Even in early pregnancy, the threads may be drawn into the uterus, so that removal becomes impossible. If the pregnancy continues to term there is no evidence of any other adverse effects.

Natural Methods

After ovulation, an egg has a lifespan of only 24 hours (and sperm can survive for up to six days in the female reproductive tract). A natural method is designed to pinpoint ovulation and will require long periods of abstinence from intercourse. Recordings of temperature, cervical mucus, and cervical palpation are often combined with calendar recordings of cycle length. In practice, the method is little used and requires a very determined couple to pursue it. Correct instruction is of paramount importance and is best obtained in a specialist family planning clinic. Supplementation with patient information leaflets is important.

Sterilisation

Male sterilisation (or vasectomy) can be carried out under a local anaesthetic, whereas female sterilisation involves a general anaesthetic. Although both have a failure rate, they are designed to have permanent effects by occluding the vas deferens in a man or the Fallopian tubes in a woman. Some GPs perform vasectomies, but in general their role is restricted to providing counselling before the procedure and then any after care that is needed. If one partner carries a risk of transmitting an inherited disease they may be the logical choice to undergo the sterilisation. If pregnancy is contraindicated in a woman, then possibly she should be offered the procedure, but her own ill health may make her more of an operative risk. For many other couples the decision will be made on the basis of personal choice.

The absence of mortality and serious morbidity with vasectomy, coupled with its better success rate, will lead many couples to opt for this technique. Studies have shown that young patients are more likely to regret sterilisation procedures, which makes surgeons reluctant to operate on this group. The couple should have reached the stage when they can never envisage wanting more children, otherwise the procedure is not for them.

Male sterilisation will not be immediately effective, as it takes time for the spermatozoa to clear from the distal portion of the vas. The time taken to achieve azoospermia relates to frequency of ejaculation. Two sperm samples should be examined after 12 and 16 weeks to confirm a successful procedure. Scrotal bruising post-operatively is common and 1–2% of men develop a painful haematoma. Local support and analgesia will be required. About 5% of men will require antibiotics for a wound infection and epididymitis is a rare complication that also requires treatment. Sperm granulomas are nodules that develop as a result of sperm leakage from the severed vas; they only require referral back to the surgeon for treatment if they are painful. In 2% of cases azoospermia is not achieved, and these men will also require review by the surgeon. Late failure as a result of recanalisation occurs rarely. The failure rate for vasectomy is 1-in-2000.

Female sterilisation is normally carried out laparoscopically by the application of clips or rings to the Fallopian tubes, and the small skin incisions are closed with absorbable sutures. There is an operative mortality, which is less than 8 per 100,000 procedures, and any post-operative discomfort should resolve within 48 hours. Technical difficulties may result in the need for a mini-laparotomy, which would be the preferred method if sterilisation is performed immediately postpartum when the uterus is large and the pelvis very vascular. There is always the possibility of bowel damage or bleeding, which should be recognised at the time of surgery. If it is not, the patient may present to the GP a few days later with abdominal pain and pyrexia and require prompt referral back to the hospital team. Female sterilisation can be carried out at the same time as pregnancy termination but is more likely to be regretted later (as is postpartum sterilisation).

It is obviously important that contraception is continued until the surgery is carried out, to ensure that the woman is not already pregnant at the time of the operation.

The procedure is effective immediately and may have no effect on menstrual cycle length and the nature of the periods. Obviously, if a woman has previously used the combined Pill, her periods will be heavier, longer, and more painful post-sterilisation; and advancing age may also produce similar effects. The failure rate of female sterilisation is 1-in-200. The woman should be counselled about the irreversibility, alternatives for contraception, the risk of ectopic pregnancy, and a 1-in-300 risk of visceral injury during the procedure.

Useful tips
○ Always have a low threshold for doing a pregnancy test.
○ If a women is having irregular vaginal bleeding exclude causes other than contraception.
○ Be wary of the woman who says no form of contraception suits her. Be prepared to discuss what is available but realise she may remain dissatisfied.

Further Reading

1. Glasier A, Gebbie A, Loudon N. *Handbook of Family Planning and Reproductive Healthcare.* [Fourth edition.] Edinburgh: Churchill Livingston, 2000.
2. Guillebaud J. *Contraception: your questions answered.* [Third Edition.] Edinburgh: Churchill Livingstone, 1999.
3. Kemmeren JM, Algra A, Grobbee DE. Third generation oral contraceptives and risk of venous thrombosis. *BMJ* 2001; **323:** 131-134.
4. Beral V, Hermon C, Kay C, *et al.* Mortality associated with oral contraceptive use: 25 year follow up of cohort of 46,000 women from Royal College of General Practitioners' Oral Contraceptive Study. *BMJ* 1999; **318:** 96-100.
5. Churchill D, Allen J, Pringle M, *et al.* Consultation patterns and provision of contraception in general practice before teenage pregnancy: case-control study. *BMJ* 2000; **321:** 486-489.
6. Jick H, Kaye JA, Vasilakis-Scarramoza C, Jick SS. Risk of venous thromboembolism among users of third generation oral contraceptives compared with users of oral contraceptives with levonorgestrel before and after 1995: cohort and case-control analysis. *BMJ* 2000; **321:** 1190-1195.
7. Harrison-Woolrych M, Duncan A, Howe J, Smith C. Improving access to emergency contraception *BMJ* 2001; **322:** 186-187.
8. Kuyoh MA, Toroitich-Ruto C, Grimes DA, *et al.* Sponge versus diaphragm for contraception (Cochrane Review). In: *The Cochrane Library,* Issue 3. Oxford: Update Software, 2002.
9. French R, Cowan F, Mansour D, *et al.* Hormonally impregnated intrauterine systems versus other forms of reversible contraceptives as effective methods of preventing pregnancy (Cochrane Review). In: *The Cochrane Library,* Issue 3. Oxford: Update Software, 2002.

Useful Websites

- http://www.ffprhc.org.uk – gives advice about training for the DFFP as well as recommendations for clinical practice
- http://www.nursingnetuk.com – gives information about family planning courses for nurses
- http://www.guidance.prodigy.nhs.uk/contraception
- http://www.fpa.org.uk – gives information for patients
- http://www.brook.org.uk – gives information for young patients

NURSE ISSUING OF HORMONAL POST-COITAL CONTRACEPTION

NURSE (or DOCTOR) _____ Date _____

Name _____ Age _____

Current Method _____

Any previous PCC? _____ If so, when? _____ Any problems with PCC? _____

Reasons for PCC:-
1. Unprotected Sexual Intercourse   ☐
2. Split Condom   ☐
3. Pill Mistakes   ☐
4. Vomiting/Diarrhoea   ☐
5. Antibiotics/Other Drug Therapy   ☐
6. Other contraceptive method problems   ☐   If so, what? _____

LMP (1st day) _____ Normal cycle is _____ Date of UPSI _____

Day of cycle   Number of hours   Any previous episodes
of UPSI _____   since UPSI _____   of UPSI in this cycle? Yes/No _____

Options explained

1. How it works   ☐
2. Side effects   ☐
3. Failure rate   ☐
4. Effects of foetus   ☐
5. How to take it   ☐
6. Follow up discussed   ☐

Current medication if any _____ BP _____

Risk of pregnancy re: ☐   IUCD option   ☐
day of cycle discussed   discussed if appropriate

PCC information   ☐
leaflet given

STATE IF PATIENT IS UNDER 16   ☐   (Gillick Competence)

Future contraception discussed   ☐   State future method if applicable

Signature _____

DOCTOR
Authorising Dr _____ via telephone/in person at _____ am/pm (delete as appropriate)
(If nurse issued)

Drs Signature _____ Date _____

Routine Antenatal and Postnatal Care

Dr Sirjit S Bath and Dr Manish Latthe

Introduction
In this chapter we will discuss some of the major issues arising when considering both antenatal and postnatal care.

Antenatal Care in General Practice
Antenatal care is provided to screen pregnancies at regular intervals in order to prevent harm to the mother and baby and achieve a successful outcome. Forms of such care have been in existence for over 50 years over which time they have greatly evolved, with the role of primary care taking the front seat. The advent of 'shared care' has significantly changed the way pregnancies are monitored and problems identified, improving care greatly and allowing hospital units to concentrate on the high-risk cases. Also, patients prefer local treatment by familiar faces to sometimes overburdened and impersonal hospitals.

The first appointment
It is usually recommended that the patient be seen before ten weeks gestation for the initial assessment. A GP, midwife, or preferably both can do this. The first hospital attendance in a low-risk pregnancy should be around 12 weeks, but many units will also perform an ultrasound scan prior to 16 weeks as part of their routine practice.

The use of standard patient-held antenatal notes has been an extremely useful advance in both the initial assessment and ongoing findings. Information that is usually to be recorded typically includes:
- age and marital status
- whether the pregnancy was planned or a failure of contraception
- LMP and EDD
- parity/gravidity
- medical and surgical history
- obstetric history
- family history (if consanguineous relationship or abnormality in first degree relative then consider genetic counselling and referral prior to 12 weeks)

- social history
- medications
- allergies
- blood group
- Rh status
- rubella immunisation.

Patient hand-held records are given to all women, usually on their first visit to the antenatal clinic. These are an important source of information to healthcare workers, as they contain information about the antenatal care of the woman. Also included is a kick chart, results of tests and scans, past medical and social history, etc. Many practices have their own equivalent maternity record card that will contain similar information but stored in the woman's medical notes in the practice.

The first visit is usually followed by an examination including:
- weight
- blood pressure
- urinalysis
- general physical examination (including cardiovascular and respiratory systems) if the patient is unknown to the GP
- abdominal – fundus if palpable
- pelvic – only done if dates are uncertain or there is pelvic pain
- cervical smear if due – though this is usually done in hospital antenatal clinic or at the postnatal visit.

Investigations are usually done following counselling at the initial visit to the hospital antenatal clinic (the booking visit). They may, however, be done in primary care if anaemia is suspected (a particular problem in Asians) or if they present to primary care late in gestation. These usually include:
- FBC
- haemoglobinopathy screen in high-risk groups
- ABO and Rh group and check for antibodies
- rubella immunity
- VDRL
- hepatitis B screen
- HIV status (opt out screening)
- screening for Down's syndrome (11–14 weeks for NT or 15–19 weeks for maternal serum screening).

With all this information at hand the GP can usually assess if the pregnancy has any risk factors of note. These must be highlighted in the referral letter to an obstetrician. Together with the parents a decision is then made about the maternity unit to be referred

to. It must be noted that some parents do prefer alternative methods of delivery and may, for example, want to be referred to a unit offering water births. Women at low risk may want to be delivered at home by their midwife or, rarely nowadays, their GP. These may include:
- second/third pregnancy in a healthy mother under 35 years
- no medical/social/psychological or obstetric complications of note.

Each request is judged on its merits and with full consultation with the mother, midwife, GP, and hospital team.

Maternal health

Health education and advice is an important part of care and usually involves diet, smoking, alcohol, dental care, and maternity benefits. Advice regarding cessation or reduction in smoking and alcohol intake must be given if necessary.

Maternal dietary advice is also important. The mother-to-be should avoid soft cheeses (though hard varieties are acceptable), liver and liver-containing foods (e.g. pâté), and raw or partially uncooked eggs (such as in mayonnaise). Also, meats should be cooked thoroughly. Adequate fluid intake must be encouraged, particularly if the woman is suffering from nausea and vomiting (e.g. due to morning sickness). A variety of patient information leaflets and booklets that deal with these and other issues during pregnancy are available (e.g. *Emma's Diary*).

The expectant mother should also be given the MatB1 form (for maternity benefits after 26 weeks) and the FW8 prescription exemption certificate form at booking; the latter lasts to 12 months after delivery.

It is recommended that women take folic acid three months prior to conception and in pregnancy up to 12 weeks gestation, as it can reduce the risk of NTDs, such as spina bifida. Current advice is that all women of childbearing age who may become pregnant should take a supplement that provides 400µg of folic acid per day. This is as well as a dietary intake of folic acid of about 200µg per day. Women with spina bifida or who have previously had an NTD-affected pregnancy should take a supplement that provides 5mg per day.

Also, relaxation classes are important and are run in local hospitals by midwives.

Pre-existing maternal medical problems

Hypertension

This should not be labelled as essential or primary hypertension until other causes of hypertension have been ruled out. The conditions to rule out include renal diseases, cardiac diseases, trophoblastic disease, phaeochromocytoma, Cushing's syndrome, and Conn's syndrome.

Pregnancies with chronic hypertension are at increased risk of:
- superimposed pre-eclampsia (five-fold increased risk)
- foetal growth restriction
- placental abruption
- increased perinatal mortality.

It is not possible to be prescriptive about the management of hypertension; for instance, the frequency and place of monitoring of blood pressure will depend on the level of hypertension, length of gestation, other prognostic factors, availability of a day care unit, and the mother's wishes. However, it is critical that hypertensive women and their foetuses have careful, well-coordinated surveillance by the community midwife, GP, and the obstetrician or obstetric physician. Management involves:
- controlling blood pressure (the commonly used antihypertensive agents in pregnancy are methyldopa, nifedipine, and labetalol; avoid ACE inhibitors)
- screening for superimposed pre-eclampsia (regular blood pressures and urinalysis) and growth restriction (fortnightly ultrasound biometry).

Pregnancy-induced hypertension without proteinuria in the second half of pregnancy and pre-eclampsia are further discussed in the chapter 'Problems in Later Pregnancy'.

Diabetes
Diabetes in pregnancy can either exist as a pre-existing condition (type 1 or 2) or, less commonly, arise during pregnancy itself (gestational diabetes). Patients with a normal glucose tolerance test but raised fasting sugar are labelled as having 'impaired fasting glaucoma' rather than gestational diabetes.

It is imperative that pre-existing diabetes should be referred to a diabetic/obstetric team for pre-pregnancy counselling. If the GP sees the woman, then it is extremely important to stress the following:
- Advise importance of planned pregnancy.
- Offer contraception until good diabetic control is achieved.
- Patients wanting to become pregnant need:
  a) rubella check
  b) preconception folic acid 400mcg daily up to the first trimester
  c) referral to diabetic clinic for assessment of treatment (e.g. insulin requirements); stop ACE inhibitors, statins, and oral diabetic therapy; improve sugar control.
- Encourage good glucose control – pre-prandial blood glucose range 3.5–5.9 and post-prandial <8mmol/l; HbA1c in upper part of normal range.
- Stop smoking and alcohol.
- When pregnancy is confirmed, arrange urgent referral to obstetrician; booking should be as soon as possible.
- Care should be hospital-based but GP can provide pre-pregnancy advice.

Diabetic control during pregnancy should be optimised. The aim is to achieve glucose concentration as near non-diabetic pregnancy levels as possible, without undue hypoglycaemia. Tight control during pregnancy reduces the risk of perinatal morbidity – neonatal hypoglycaemia, neonatal hyperbilirubinaemia, macrosomia – and neonatal mortality.

Gestational diabetes mellitus is a type of diabetes that arises during pregnancy (usually during the second or third trimester).

If glycosuria (++ or more) is present during routine antenatal visits, the woman should have a random blood sugar test performed or an oral glucose tolerance test (which is preferred by some departments). This will confirm if diabetes or impaired glucose tolerance is present. A normal glucose tolerance test in the early part of pregnancy does not itself establish that GDM may not develop later. Formal systematic testing for GDM is usually done between 24 and 28 weeks of gestation.

Risk factors associated with GDM
○ Previous GDM
○ Obesity
○ Family history of diabetes
○ Unexplained stillbirth in a previous pregnancy
○ Previous baby >4kg
○ Polyhydramnios
○ Large for gestational age foetus in current pregnancy

Treatment of GDM:
- Often dietary control is all that is necessary.
- Blood glucose target levels are the same as for women with type 1 or type 2 diabetes.
- If blood sugar levels are consistently above the target levels then insulin should be started under specialist care. Insulin can usually be stopped after delivery.
- If blood glucose control is good, then the woman can receive the same care during labour and delivery as any woman without diabetes.

Useful tips
○ The prevalence of GDM is higher in ethnic minority populations.
○ The importance of diagnosing GDM relates to the high risk of future diabetes and to the risk of macrosomia and intrauterine death in severe cases.
○ Management of GDM is with diet in the first instance, followed by insulin in resistant cases. GDM is best handled in a joint obstetrics–diabetology clinic with dedicated experts.

○ Pregnancy and puerperium provide a unique opportunity for education regarding lifestyle and dietary changes.

Others

• *Asthma.* Pregnancy itself does not influence the severity of asthma. Treatment of asthma in pregnancy does not differ from its management in non-pregnant women. Education and reassurance, ideally preconception, concerning the safety of asthma medication during pregnancy are integral parts of management.

• *Epilepsy.* Most anticonvulsant drugs are teratogenic. Monotherapy is better than polytherapy. All women taking anticonvulsants should receive pre-pregnancy counselling (and should discuss with their specialist the need for continuing therapy) and be given folic acid 5mg daily preconceptually and throughout pregnancy. Breastfeeding while taking anticonvulsants is safe.

Screening for Down's syndrome

At the time of writing, about 80% of pregnant women in the UK are offered non-invasive Down's syndrome screening. However, there are wide variations in the screening tests offered. By 2004, the UK NSC aims for all pregnant women to be offered the option of non-invasive tests for Down's syndrome, which would reduce the number of unnecessary amniocentesis tests.

The most widely used tests depend on measuring biochemical markers in the maternal blood, in conjunction with the maternal age. These markers are AFP, uE3, inhibin-A (inhibin), and free b-hCG. These tests are performed between 15 and 19 weeks of gestation. A raised level of AFP is associated with an increased risk of having a pregnancy with an open NTD, abdominal wall defect, or IUGR. AFP is low in Down's syndrome and other autosomal trisomies.

The current advice of the NSC on Down's syndrome screening recommends that all pregnant women should be offered second trimester serum screening based on the measurement of at least two biochemical markers, with a risk of greater than 1-in-250–350 to be considered an increased risk. Screen-positive women as well as women over 35 years of age on the EDD are offered further tests, such as amniocentesis or CVS.

There are many problems with current screening. Firstly, as maternal age increases, any relative benefit of the biochemical tests over age-related screening decreases. Secondly, cost-benefit is debatable; benefits depend on a high uptake of amniocentesis and termination. Thirdly, the biochemical levels have not been determined for ethnic minority populations and therefore these tests are less useful for them (they will have a higher false positive rate). Fourthly, screening can cause a great deal of distress – counselling for

Down's screening is time consuming and it is not easy for most parents-to-be to understand all of the relevant issues. Proper consent for screening tests and their implications is a controversial area.

An alternative to measuring biochemical markers is high-resolution ultrasound at around 10–14 weeks to measure foetal NT. There is a strong association between increased foetal NT and chromosome abnormality, as well as heart defects.

It seems that in the future, first trimester maternal serum screening with NT (between 11 and 13^{+6}) and added second trimester serum screening to reduce the false positive rate has the potential to detect over 80% of Down's syndrome foetuses in early pregnancy with a false positive rate of 1%. The cost implications of this mean that it may not become adopted everywhere.

A recent retrospective audit of different antenatal screening policies for Down's syndrome in eight district general hospitals found that serum screening and nuchal scanning did not achieve significantly higher antenatal detection rates of Down's syndrome than the use of maternal age and routine anomaly scanning. The authors of this study believed that this was because the initial statistical models of screening used the wrong assumptions. This field of obstetrics is constantly changing.

The standard method of antenatal diagnosis of Down's syndrome is amniocentesis between 15–18 weeks of pregnancy, followed by karyotyping of cultured cells from the amniotic fluid. The excess foetal loss attributed to amniocentesis is about 0.5–1%. Earlier diagnosis can be achieved by transabdominal CVS. It is less accurate than amniocentesis and there is a 1–2% risk of miscarriage, however earlier terminations are associated with a lower morbidity than later terminations.

Antenatal surveillance
The GP and/or midwife typically see the patient every four weeks up to 28 weeks, then fortnightly until 36 weeks, followed by weekly until term. If needed, care is then taken over by the hospital and specialist. This, however, is dependent on each individual case and acts only as a guideline.

Standard assessments include:
- blood pressure
- urinalysis
- weight
- fundal height (preferably in centimetres above the symphysis pubis)
- checking for peripheral oedema
- foetal heart (after about 15–20 weeks and preferably with sonicaid)
- foetal lie and presentation (after second trimester)

- blood tests (FBC and Rh antibodies at 34 weeks in all pregnant women, Rh antibodies are also checked at 28 weeks in Rh-negative women). In some regions there is routine anti-D prophylaxis at 28 and/or 34 weeks for Rh-negative women. Routine anti-D prophylaxis at 28 and 34 weeks is recommend for all Rh-negative women by NICE but many disagree with this view, including the Royal College of Midwives and many consultant obstetricians.

If there are any problems, the hospital day care units can usually review the patient at short notice. Here, women with problems like mild-moderate pre-eclampsia, growth restriction, cholestasis, and similar problems can now be managed on an outpatient basis.

Conditions that may need referral to hospital include:
- high blood pressure with or without oedema/headaches (risk of pre-eclampsia)
- proteinuria (pre-eclampsia)
- vaginal bleeding (placental abruption/praevia)
- glycosuria (occult or pregnancy-induced diabetes)
- recurrent UTIs
- oligohydramnios (IUGR)
- polyhydramnios (foetal malformations/diabetes)
- small-for-dates uterus (risk of IUGR)
- large-for-dates uterus (risk of macrosomia)
- reduced foetal movements (risk of foetal compromise)
- malpresentation (after 36 weeks).

Postnatal Care in General Practice
After childbirth, the mother's physiology and anatomy returns to normal. This period is referred to as the puerperium. There is recent evidence that short-term postnatal morbidity is extensive and that many of these problems can become chronic.

Lactation
Following birth, hormonal triggers are released to commence lactation. This is mediated by neuro-endocrine pathways such that suckling at the nipple releases breast milk and stimulates further production. There is no doubt that breast milk improves the health of newborn babies in many ways, including:
- boosts the immune system
- lowers incidence of autoimmune disorders
- reduces risk of cot death
- reduces neonatal seizures
- reduces gastro-intestinal problems
- improves bonding.

Lactation also provides some contraceptive protection (though this is not reliable).

Sometimes suppression of lactation is needed with bromocriptin; for example, after neonatal death. Breast engorgement can be a problem and is usually relieved with proper bra support and analgesia.

Mastitis

While breasts can become very inflamed and sore, they rarely develop an abscess formation. Mastitis can be due to failure of milk expression from a lobule, and helping the baby to empty the breast and cold compresses are effective. Mastitis may be complicated by *Staphylococcus aureus* infection when treatment with flucloxacillin is usually given. If a breast abscess is formed then incision and drainage is needed. The best treatment is to continue breastfeeding (or expression) from the breast affected, as this should relieve any duct blockage and therefore treat the mastitis.

As many as two-thirds of women report problems with breastfeeding, including nipple pain, engorgement, cracks, and bleeding. Proper advice and counselling is usually all that is needed.

Secondary postpartum haemorrhage

Secondary postpartum haemorrhage occurs where there is a significant blood loss between 24 hours and six weeks after delivery. The commonest causes are retained fragments of placenta, blood clot, or infection. If the bleeding is not excessive and there are no systemic signs of infection, the patient may be treated at home with antibiotics and analgesia. If, however, the bleeding is significant and there are systemic signs, the patient will need an urgent ultrasound scan. The uterus may also be palpably large and tender. A uterine evacuation under general anaesthetic and antibiotic cover will be needed to remove the retained products.

Estimates of postnatal anaemia of about 25–30% suggest that its diagnosis and treatment is important.

Puerperal pyrexia

Puerperal pyrexia is defined as a temperature of 38°C or above during the first 14 days post-delivery. Infection of the urinary or genital tract must be excluded, as must mastitis and respiratory infection. Appropriate antibiotics are then used as necessary. Preventing or reducing the predisposing factors is very important (postpartum infections are less frequent today than in the past because of better aseptic techniques). A fever that occurs between days 4 and 10 postpartum and that does not respond to antibiotics may indicate developing pelvic thrombophlebitis, which should be managed in the usual way as for thrombosis.

Postnatal depression

While some emotional lability after birth is not uncommon (sometimes called 'baby blues'), between 10–15% of women experience postnatal depression, which may occur up to one year after delivery. The cause of postnatal depression is not clear; possibly involved are changes in hormone levels during the postpartum period. Personality and psychoanalytic theories also exist, and social factors may be important. Factors associated with postnatal depression include: previous psychiatric disorder (e.g. previous depression or anxiety), obstetric complications, age, parity, marriage or relationship problems, social class, housing problems, social or psychological stress, unplanned pregnancy, and being unmarried.

Symptoms, often disabling, include fatigue, insomnia, inability to cope, and suicidal thoughts. Health visitors do a depression score if alerted to the problem and this will identify significant cases. For such women, antidepressant therapy should be commenced and involvement of the local psychiatric services sought urgently, as supportive counselling has been found to be beneficial. Care of the baby must also be shared among close relatives. In extreme cases, postnatal psychosis is seen; the mother becomes delusional and even violent and may need to be sectioned for the sake of baby and mother. This can recur in subsequent pregnancies and such cases need to be monitored by psychiatrists with a special interest in postnatal depression.

Postnatal visits

Currently, GPs are able to claim a fee for completing up to five home visits in the first 14 postnatal days. Most GPs do not do the full five visits, as a midwife normally visits the mother frequently during this period also. During these visits, the GP will examine the mother (e.g. to check for suture healing or to assess blood pressure) and do a routine postnatal examination for the baby. It is an opportunity to address any concerns that the parents have (e.g. feeding problems) and to discuss contraception if appropriate.

The postnatal examination

This is usually performed at six weeks and should include:
- blood pressure
- urinalysis
- weight
- contraceptive advice
- pelvic examination
- cervical smear if needed.

This is usually complemented by advice on pelvic floor exercises and discussion about future pregnancies if needed. If the woman complains of urinary or faecal incontinence, then she should be referred to the physiotherapist.

Useful tips
○ Pregnancy often puts a great deal of stress on the pregnant woman and her family, and this should be recognised and treated appropriately.
○ Shared care only works effectively when primary care physicians access secondary care sooner rather than later if any deviations from the norm are found.

○ Effective antenatal clinics can only be achieved by teamwork and sharing with midwives, doctors, and ancillary staff.

Further Reading

1. Chamberlain G (ed). *Turnbull's Obstetrics.* [2nd ed.] Edinburgh: Churchill Livingstone, 1995.
2. Pearson V. *Frequency and timing of antenatal visits.* Bristol: Healthcare Evaluation Unit, University of Bristol, 1994.
3. Sikorski J, Wilson J, Clement S, *et al.* A randomised controlled trial comparing two schedules of antenatal visits: the antenatal care project. *BMJ* 1996; **312:** 546-553.
4. Villar J, Carroli G, Khan-Neelofur D, *et al.* Patterns of routine antenatal care for low-risk pregnancy (Cochrane Review). In: *The Cochrane Library,* Issue 2. Oxford: Update Software, 2002.
5. Ackermann-Liebrich U, Voegli T, Guenther-Witt K, *et al.* Home versus hospital deliveries: a prospective study on matched pairs. *BMJ* 1996; **313:** 1313-1318.
6. National Institute for Clinical Excellence. *Technology Appraisal Guidance No. 41. Routine antenatal anti-D prophylaxis for RhD-negative women.* Issue Date: March-April 2002. Review Date: March 2005.
7. MRC Vitamin Study Research Group. Prevention of neural tube defects: results of the Medical Research Council vitamin study. *Lancet* 1991; **338:** 131-137.
8. Lumley J, Watson L, Watson M, Bower C. Periconceptional supplementation with folate and/or multivitamins for preventing neural tube defects (Cochrane Review). In: *The Cochrane Library,* Issue 2. Oxford: Update Software, 2002.
9. Wellesley D, Boyle T, Barber J, Howe DT. Retrospective audit of different antenatal screening policies for Down's syndrome in eight district general hospitals in one health region. *BMJ* 2002; **325:** 15.
10. Evans J, Heron J, Francomb H, *et al.* Cohort study of depressed mood during pregnancy and after childbirth. *BMJ* 2001; **323:** 257-260.

Useful Websites

- The Fetal Medicine Foundation is a charity that promotes research and training in foetal medicine. URL: http://www.fetalmedicine.com/.
- Antenatal Results and Choices. ARC is the only national charity that provides non-directive support and information to parents throughout the antenatal testing process. URL: http://www.arc-uk.org.
- The Down's Syndrome Association. URL: http://www.downs-syndrome.org.uk.
- Association for Spina Bifida and Hydrocephalus. URL: http://www.asbah.demon.co.uk.
- *Emma's Diary.* This step-by-step guide to pregnancy is produced by the RCGP. *Emma's Diary* is updated every six months and is given to women at the start of their pregnancy. URL: http://www.rcgp.org.uk/rcgp/publications/em_diary.asp.

Problems in Early Pregnancy

Dr Sirjit S Bath and Dr Manish Latthe

Introduction
In this chapter we discuss problems in pregnancy before the gestational age of viability. Women with problems in early pregnancy will usually seek the help of their GP. The commonest problem is miscarriage. The other common problems are morning sickness, fatigue, and pelvic pain.

Miscarriage
Miscarriage (abortion) is defined as expulsion or extraction of a foetus or embryo weighing 500g or less and/or less than 24 weeks gestation. Miscarriage occurs in about 15% of confirmed pregnancies.

The loss of a wanted pregnancy is always distressing to the mother irrespective of the timing. More pregnancies are lost in the first trimester than in the other two trimesters. We will not discuss termination of pregnancy in this chapter.

Spontaneous miscarriage
Spontaneous miscarriage may be threatened, inevitable, incomplete, complete, or missed. Patients almost invariably ask their GP for the cause of their loss. Understandably, this is a time of distressing emotions and words must be spoken with great care and thought. In most cases, no explanation for the miscarriage can be determined. A high proportion of spontaneous miscarriages (over 90%) are thought to result from the abnormal development of the foetus. This can manifest as blighted ovum, which is an empty sac in which the embryo has not developed beyond a small clump of cells. Other factors that can be implicated include:
- chromosomal abnormalities
- structural or genetic anomalies
- placental failure
- multiple pregnancy
- infections
- endocrine disorders; e.g. polycystic ovaries, luteal phase defect
- immunological causes.

Around 85% of spontaneous miscarriages occur in the first trimester; those occurring in the second trimester are usually from maternal causes, such as:
- incompetent cervix
- congenital or acquired anomalies of the uterine cavity
- endocrine (hypothyroidism, diabetes mellitus)
- chronic disorders like nephritis, etc.
- acute infections, including viral (e.g. rubella)
- immunological causes
- major physical trauma.

Threatened miscarriage
- This is the commonest presentation faced by a GP. There is usually a period of amenorrhoea followed by vaginal bleeding.
- Characteristically, it is associated with little or no pain.
- There is no evidence-based data to show that bed rest improves the outcome, but most GPs feel that it is sensible to advise the patient not to overexert herself.
- An early USS can usually be arranged on the same or next day as diagnosis in most hospitals now. The development of the early pregnancy assessment unit can be hailed as one of the great innovations in the handling of early pregnancy problems for patients. If the scan demonstrates a foetal heart, there is at least a 90% chance that the pregnancy will reach the gestational age of viability. There is a less than 2% chance of miscarriage with ultrasound evidence of live foetus at eight to ten weeks, and a <1% chance of miscarriage with ultrasound evidence of live foetus at more than ten weeks gestation.

Inevitable miscarriage
- This is characterised by amenorrhoea followed by heavy bleeding with clots and pain. In extreme cases there may be products of conception passing into the vagina.
- This can be an emergency, as collapse can occur due to excessive bleeding. The patient's vital signs, therefore, should be measured and intravenous access obtained if possible. Pain relief may also be needed. The patient must be suitably transported to an alerted gynaecologist at the nearest hospital.
- An evacuation of the uterus under general anaesthetic is performed if the woman is bleeding heavily, a procedure termed 'evacuation of the retained products of conception'.

Incomplete miscarriage
- Persistence of products of conception inside the uterine cavity on transvaginal scan merits evacuation if the patient is symptomatic in the form of persistent vaginal bleeding or has foul smelling discharge with pyrexia (infection). It is preferable to commence antibiotics prior to the procedure.

- If this is suspected by the GP, then immediate referral to secondary care is required.

Complete miscarriage
- Amenorrhoea is followed by a variable amount of bleeding, which has usually stopped when the woman presents for consultation.
- The uterus is smaller than expected for the length of amenorrhoea.

Missed miscarriage
- This occurs when the pregnancy has failed but the products are retained in the uterus.
- There is usually a period of amenorrhoea during which minimal vaginal bleeding may have occurred.
- The patient may confirm that she does not feel pregnant and early pregnancy symptoms may indeed have diminished or gone.
- The patient should be referred to the early pregnancy assessment unit. In early pregnancy with empty gestational sac <4ml in volume or when foetal pole is seen without foetal heart (<6mm), a repeat transvaginal scan is arranged in seven to ten days. If the sac is over 6mm and there is absence of foetal heart, missed miscarriage is confirmed.
- Empty gestation sac with volume >4ml or diameter >20mm confirms blighted ovum.
- The options of management, i.e. medical or surgical treatment, are discussed with the patient. Surgical management is in the form of suction–evacuation of the uterus. Mifepristone followed by vaginal or oral prostaglandins achieves complete evacuation of the uterus in 90–95% of cases.
- The option of conservative management (awaiting events) is preferred by a minority of patients. The patient is advised to return to the hospital if the pain or bleeding becomes excessive. The patient is given contact details if any concerns arise or alternatively, a rescan can be arranged in seven to ten days to rule out retained products of conception.
- The importance of psychological support for a woman undergoing this traumatic episode in her life cannot be underestimated.

Recurrent miscarriages
- Sadly, about 1% of women in the reproductive age experience three or more consecutive miscarriages. It is useful, however, to reassure patients, as the spontaneous chance of a subsequent successful pregnancy is around 75%.
- These pregnancies, however, do need careful monitoring, as there is a higher chance of other pregnancy complications.
- There are many causes of recurrent miscarriage:
  a) genetic factors; e.g. chromosomal abnormality

  b) anatomical factors; e.g. uterine structural abnormalities
  c) cervical incompetence
  d) endocrine factors; e.g. inadequate secretion of progesterone during the early
     weeks of pregnancy; diabetes mellitus and thyroid disease; hypersecretion of LH
     as in polycystic ovarian disease (found in 50% of women with recurrent
     miscarriage)
  e) autoimmune factors; e.g. primary antiphospholipid syndrome has 90%
     miscarriage rate when they receive no treatment
  f) thrombophilic defects – the current treatment used is either low dose aspirin
     (75mg daily) or aspirin in combination with heparin
  g) infections – unclear if they can cause recurrent miscarriage; bacterial vaginosis
     has been implicated in a few studies.
- These patients are usually investigated in a pre-pregnancy clinic to try to identify
  and correct possible causes. Referral and investigation usually takes place after the
  third miscarriage or sometimes earlier if, for example, the patient wishes it.
- Support from friends and family is also very important for women with recurrent
  miscarriage in whom no cause for the miscarriages is identified.

Septic abortion
- This is abortion complicated by infection of the uterine contents.
- This presents as an incomplete abortion associated with systemic signs of sepsis.
  Rarely, this may be due to amateur attempts at procuring an abortion.
- The infection is usually mild but can spread to the uterine wall in 15% of cases and
  rarely can cause shock and disseminated intravascular coagulation.
- Treatment is by antibiotics orally or intravenous depending on the severity. As in
  most cases, *E.coli*, streptococci, and/or anaerobes are implicated; metronidazole with
  a broad-spectrum antibiotic is the treatment of choice.
- Evacuation is usually done when the patient has stabilised and has had parenteral
  antibiotics for about 12 hours.

Ectopic pregnancy
Ectopic pregnancy is defined as the implantation of a pregnancy outside the uterine cavity.
The commonest site is in the Fallopian tubes, accounting for 95% of cases. The incidence
is about 24 per 1000 pregnancies and 65% occur between 25–34 years of age. The risk of
recurrence is in the order of 10–20%. This is a serious condition and can be associated with
maternal death.

Diagnosis
- Ectopic pregnancies are notorious for not presenting with classical symptoms.
  However, they should be considered when there is a history of a missed period
  associated with unilateral lower abdominal pain and occasionally some vaginal
  spotting. Occasionally, the history of amenorrhoea cannot be elicited.

- On examination the uterus may be enlarged with cervical excitation. One side of the uterus may also be tender associated with a palpable mass. Vaginal examination must always be done with care, as tubal rupture can be precipitated. In advanced cases shoulder tip pain can be caused by bleeding and diaphragmatic irritation.

Investigation
- For patients who are clinically stable, monoclonal antibody tests for b-hCG are done. If urine testing is positive, a serum assay is done. Most women with an ectopic pregnancy have a serum level less than 3000 U/L. The rate of rise is also helpful. A doubling time of around two days may suggest a normally located pregnancy. A negative serum result rules out an ectopic pregnancy.
- The clinical picture, however, is important and a period of observation may be prudent in these cases. The levels of b-hCG rise slower if the pregnancy is outside the uterus. If tests are positive but the pregnancy cannot be located by ultrasound, they need to be repeated in 48 hours.
- The definitive diagnostic aid is a laparoscopy, although very early cases can be missed.

Management
- The woman should be referred to the early pregnancy assessment unit on the same day for appropriate investigations and prompt management.
- If the patient is shocked, emergency transportation to hospital is mandatory. Intravenous access and resuscitation should be done while waiting. At hospital immediate laparotomy is usually performed in order to arrest the haemorrhage and stabilise the patient.
- If the patient is haemodynamically stable, laparoscopic surgery by a fully trained surgeon is the approach of choice. A salpingectomy is usually performed. Salpingostomy is usually not performed because of the high risk of recurrence.
- Before proceeding to laparoscopy, however, caution must be observed in cases of marked obesity or significant haematosalpinx or haemorrhage. It may also be difficult in patients with pelvic adhesions or a cornual pregnancy. Following conservative surgery, b-hCG levels in the blood are monitored to exclude persistent trophoblast.
- Intratubal injection of methotrexate (if there is no haemoperitoneum) under laparoscopic or ultrasonic guidance is significantly less successful in eliminating tubal pregnancy.
- Methotrexate is an alternative option in a selected group after counselling regarding the benefits and risks.
- Other sites of ectopic pregnancy are rare and include cornual, ovarian, abdominal, and cervical. These are usually discovered by ultrasound or laparoscopy, although cases of abdominal pregnancy may only be diagnosed when the patient presents with acute abdominal pain in the second/third trimester.

Hyperemesis gravidarum
- Nausea is common up to 16 weeks. Anti-emetics appear to reduce the frequency of nausea in early pregnancy, although there is some concern about adverse effects, but there is no evidence of foetal damage.
- Hyperemesis gravidarum occurs when the usual sickness in pregnancy becomes persistent and severe. It affects 1–2% of pregnancies and is characterised by dehydration (weight loss of 5% or more, reduced urine output, and loss of skin turgor), electrolyte disturbance, and ketosis. If left untreated, it can lead to CNS damage, liver and renal failure, and ultimately death. Fortunately, these extreme cases rarely occur in modern practice.
- The onset is around six to eight weeks gestation, but the diagnosis is one of exclusion. New symptoms appearing after 12 weeks gestation should not be attributed to hyperemesis gravidarum.
- There are numerous themes that are common factors and may be implicated in the underlying aetiology. It is commoner in:
  a) primigravidae
  b) multiple pregnancy
  c) molar pregnancy
  d) patients with a history of previous hyperemesis.
- The vomiting centre of some patients may also be more sensitive, as in travel sickness. The actual causal agent has not been identified, but it is thought that oestrogen is implicated in view of its effects in the Pill, although b-hCG has also been implicated. Interestingly, patients with no nausea and vomiting have a higher risk of abortion and premature labour, presumably due to lower levels of oestrogen.

Management
- Mild cases can be managed at home with oral rehydration and anti-emetics complemented with dietary advice. Anti-emetic medication appears to reduce the frequency of nausea in early pregnancy. The anti-emetics that can be taken as required and are safe in the first trimester include: prochlorperazine 5mg po tds, cyclizine 50mg po tds, metoclopramide 10mg po tds, etc.
- Of newer treatments, pyridoxine (vitamin B6) appears to be more effective in reducing the severity of nausea. The results from trials of P6 acupressure are equivocal. The results of the trial using adrenocorticotropic hormone to treat hyperemesis gravidarum show no evidence of benefit. Ginger may be of benefit, but the evidence so far is weak.
- If this fails and there are signs of dehydration, hospital care is mandatory. In hospital the patient is rehydrated with intravenous fluid therapy and parenteral anti-emetics. In most cases one or two days of this therapy is sufficient. Renal function tests (urea and electrolytes) and MSU must be done. USS is done to exclude multiple or molar pregnancy. If the patient fails to respond, other diagnoses must be considered; thyroid function tests should be done to exclude thyrotoxicosis. Other possible

diagnoses include surgical causes (appendix, obstruction, ovarian cyst), raised intracranial pressure, or metabolic dysfunction (diabetes, hypercalcaemia). Rarely, termination is necessary for life-threatening dehydration and ketosis.

Gestational trophoblastic disease and hydatidiform moles

- The development of hydatidiform moles is rare and occurs in about 1-in-1200 pregnancies.
- Clinicians are usually alerted by the symptoms of excessive b-hCG. These include amenorrhoea associated with severe pregnancy symptoms such as hyperemesis. There may be irregular bleeding or incomplete miscarriage. Pre-eclampsia may occur earlier than usual. Rarely, it may be associated with hyperthyroidism or even trophoblastic embolisation and respiratory symptoms. It is commoner at the extremes of reproductive age (over 40 or under 15), multiple pregnancy, and previous molar pregnancy. It is usually picked up at ultrasound where there is the typical 'snow storm' appearance. The b-hCG levels may also be very high.
- Very rarely, the mole may invade the myometrium or even present in the placenta, in which cases hysterectomy is usually required.
- Choriocarcinoma can occur within two years of a mole (1-in-30 cases). The disease is usually managed successfully with chemotherapy and subsequent pregnancies are mostly normal.

Management
- Suction curettage is the method of choice of evacuation for complete molar pregnancies. In complete molar pregnancies, medical termination and pre-operative cervical preparation is avoided. In partial molar pregnancies where size of foetal parts deters suction curettage, medical termination can be used.
- The RCOG and DoH have agreed that registration of women with a molar pregnancy is desirable. Women with the following molar pregnancies should be registered: complete H. mole, partial H. mole, twin pregnancy with a complete or partial H. mole, and limited macroscopic or microscopic molar change judged to require follow-up. The screening centres judge the duration of follow-up.
- Screening centres in the UK are based at Charing Cross Hospital, London; Weston Park Hospital, Sheffield; and Ninewells Hospital, Dundee.
- Women should be advised not to conceive until they have had six months of normal b-hCG. After conclusion of any further pregnancy, at any gestation, further samples are requested to rule out recurrence (1:74).
- The COCP as well as HRT can be used after b-hCG levels return to normal.

Minor Disorders of Pregnacy

Although these may be deemed trivial, they can cause great concern to patients and are very commonly presented to the health professional. Reassurance is usually all that is required but is necessary in most cases. The introduction of simple booklets given on the first antenatal visit has proved very useful in helping pregnant patients understand what is normal and symptoms that do require a medical opinion.

Morning sickness

- 70–80% of pregnant women experience nausea of some degree during the first trimester, and approximately half will actually vomit.
- It is usually worse on awakening in the morning and aggravated by the smell of food or cooking. This can of course lead to hyperemesis, as discussed previously.
- It is advised to have frequent small meals, avoiding fatty or spicy foods. Occasionally, anti-emetics are required.
- Oral fluid intake should be encouraged to prevent dehydration.
- It is very important, however, to reassure the patient that it is very common in early pregnancy and usually self-limiting.

Headache

- This is a common complaint and is thought to be due to the increase in haemodynamic volume and intravascular changes related to steroid hormones. It usually passes after the first trimester but in some patients may persist throughout pregnancy. Paracetamol and rest is advised, but investigation may be required if attacks are severe and persistent or associated with any neurological signs.

Fainting

- This is probably related to general vasodilatation associated with progesterone, which occurs before the blood volume has increased to adequate levels. Reassurance and avoiding hot atmospheres are required. Hypotension must also be excluded.

Fatigue

- This probably reflects the major physiological changes that are occurring. This may be associated with breathlessness probably related to expanding of pulmonary vasculature. After excluding any underlying cause such as anaemia, rest and a good diet are recommended.

Frequency

- Frequency of micturition is one of the symptoms of early pregnancy and probably reflects a combination of pressure on the bladder by the enlarging uterus and an increased amount of urine due to an increased blood flow and glomerular filtration. If associated with dysuria, however, cystitis must be excluded. This may also lead to insomnia.

Vaginal discharge

- Most commonly, this is due to vaginal candidiasis, but other infections do occur, such as bacterial vaginosis. In practice, most GPs will treat for candida (e.g. with a course of clotrimazole pessaries) and if that is ineffective, will then take a high vaginal swab. A watery discharge may be liquor; if this is suspected on speculum examination, a high vaginal swab is sent for microscopy and culture and immediate referral for an obstetric assessment is done. The use of nitrazine paper to detect amniotic fluid is unreliable due to the high false positive rate.

Useful tips
○ If a USS is preformed on a woman suffering with bleeding in early pregnancy and an 'empty uterus' is found, this could be due to an intrauterine pregnancy that is too early to detect, as well as an ectopic pregnancy or a complete miscarriage.
○ A positive pregnancy test in the presence of an IUCD or sterilisation must be viewed with great suspicion, as there is a greatly increased risk of ectopic pregnancy.
○ Rh-negative women who suffer a miscarriage or ectopic pregnancy will require anti-D prophylaxis.
○ Treat newly pregnant patients with extra sympathy, as they are usually emotionally labile and under stress from family and work. Of course, any complication can be devastating.
○ Loss of a pregnancy can have the same effect as any bereavement for the prospective parents, and may need to be treated as such. They can be referred for counselling if necessary, and put in touch with the appropriate support groups.

Infections in Pregnancy
Treatment for these disorders is usually in secondary care. Urgent referral by the GP is essential if a potentially serious maternal infection occurs during pregnancy.

The foetus has very little IgM or IgA until the second half of pregnancy, and no effective IgG or cell-mediated immunity until after birth. Transplacental immunoglobulins provide passive immunity against those infections to which the mother is immune, and breastfeeding maintains this cover until the baby's immune system matures. Infections affecting the foetus occur either from primary infections of the mother and then placental infection or, less often, are acquired perinatally by the foetus as it passes through the birth canal. Breast milk transmission occurs with some infections; e.g. CMV and HIV. Neonatal tetanus may be contracted via the umbilical cord stump.

Chickenpox
This is a common problem that presents to GPs. There are two times when maternal infection is a problem:
1. Before 20 weeks – risk of foetal varicella syndrome; this is relatively rare (1–2%). In the case of primary infection before 20 weeks, a detailed USS at 20 weeks to rule out anomalies will reassure parents.

2. The mother develops a rash within a week before delivery to a month afterwards. It takes about a week for the mother to pass on the antibody immunity to the baby. Thus, if the baby is born before that time, it is at risk of overwhelming infection after birth.

However, if the mother has definitely had chickenpox before, there is no risk to the foetus or neonate. To assess immunity, IgG levels for varicella can be checked. Varicella zoster immunoglobulin therapy can then be given if required, though it will not be effective if the chickenpox contact was more than ten days prior.

Rubella
Rubella is rarely a problem now because of vaccination. First trimester infection can cause congenital rubella syndrome, whose prominent features include:
- low birth weight, FTT, increased mortality
- microcephaly and mental retardation
- microphthalmia and cataracts
- deafness and malformation of organ of Corti
- patent ductus arteriosus, patent intraventricular septum
- hepatosplenomegaly, thrombocytopaenia, anaemia.

Routine antenatal screening detects those requiring puerperal vaccination. Non-immunised women should avoid pregnancy for three months, as the vaccine is a live vaccine.

Cytomegalovirus
Maternal CMV infection is very often subclinical. Diagnosis is by serology. Most congenitally infected children are asymptomatic. The symptomatic infant is characteristically born with a petechial rash, hepatosplenomegaly, jaundice, inflammation of the retina, intracranial calcifications, and microcephaly. Only about 1-in-10 infants congenitally infected with CMV has these symptoms. Long-term complications are deafness and learning difficulties.

Parvovirus B19
There is minimal risk to the foetus if the infection is caught after the pregnancy has reached 20 weeks, but before 20 weeks there is an extra 9% risk of miscarriage and a 3% risk of hydrops foetalis (the foetus develops anaemia and heart failure). There is no evidence that parvovirus B19 infection causes birth defects or learning difficulties.

Syphilis
This affects about 1-in-3500 antenatal patients. Infection during pregnancy causes congenital syphilis syndrome: rhinitis, hepatosplenomegaly and lymphadenopathy, abnormalities of bones, teeth and cartilage, and saddle nose. Nearly half of all infected infants die shortly before or after birth.

Maternal sexually transmitted disease prevention advice is important. If maternal infection occurs or is detected during pregnancy, it should be treated as soon as possible, which will prevent vertical transmission; e.g. procaine benzylpenicillin (750mg daily by intramuscular injection).

Toxoplasma

Foetal infection can occur when a pregnant mother has primary infection or occasionally with a recurrent infection. Maternal infection is mild and sometimes subclinical. Pregnant women who have cats as pets may increase their risk of developing toxoplasmosis and should not handle the litter. Infection early in pregnancy results in more severe problems than later infection. Congenital toxoplasmosis is characterised by damage to the eyes, nervous system, skin, and ears, and may result in:

- miscarriage, stillbirth, or survival with growth problems
- microcephaly and hepatosplenomegaly
- neonatal period – convulsions, jaundice, chorioretinitis, hydrocephaly, and learning difficulties
- 15% foetal damage or death in first trimester, but 60% in third trimester.

If a woman is found to have acquired toxoplasmosis during pregnancy, she should have a detailed USS and serial growth scans. After 20 weeks gestation, she may be offered cordocentesis, which is the definitive test.

Perinatal infections

Chlamydia and gonorrhoea infections can cause eye infections in the baby by being passed on at delivery. Chlamydia (can cause neonatal pneumonia also) affects about 5% of pregnancies; gonorrhoea (causes ophthalmia neonatorum) is much rarer. The mother must be reassessed after pregnancy to check that her infection has been cleared. Both infections can be treated during pregnancy. Referral to genito-urinary medicine clinic for treatment and contact screening is the usual management. Treatment during pregnancy for Chlamydia: erythromycin is used or amoxicillin 500mg tds orally for one week. *Chlamydia trachomatis* is associated with low birth weight, premature rupture of membranes, and foetal death. One-in-three infected mothers has affected babies.

Herpes simplex infection is usually acquired at birth when the mother has active cervical lesions; in this case, Caesarean section is advised. If the lesions are inactive, the baby can be delivered vaginally. Infected neonates should be isolated and treated with acyclovir, under specialist care.

In the UK, there are <1% carriers of hepatitis B. Hepatitis B infection is also usually a perinatal infection; persistent infection is very common (infected males' lifetime risk of developing hepatocellular cancer is 50%, females' is 20%). Most will develop cirrhosis. Immunisation is recommended: neonates of known carriers should receive hepatitis B immunoglobulin (0.5ml IM within 12 hours of birth), and hepatitis B vaccine (0.5ml IM within seven days and at one and six months).

Testing for HIV infection is routine in some hospitals, especially in high-risk areas. HIV infection passes to the baby in about 15% of cases but is reduced to 8% with anti-retroviral drug treatment (zidovudine) during delivery and elective Caesarean section. With appropriate management, infected mothers are unlikely to give birth to infected children. The DoH recommends that all women under NHS care should be offered antenatal testing. All infected women should receive anti-retroviral treatment during the third trimester and labour, with their babies receiving the drug for the first six weeks of life.

Further Reading

1. Zhang W, Wang L. Mifepristone in treating ectopic pregnancy. *Chin Med J (Engl)* 1999; **112(4):** 376-378.
2. Jewell D, Young G. Interventions for nausea and vomiting in early pregnancy (Cochrane Review). In: *The Cochrane Library,* Issue 1. Oxford: Update Software, 2002.
3. Disorders of early pregnancy (ectopic, miscarriage, GTD). In: Campbell S, Monga A (eds). *Gynaecology by Ten Teachers.* [17th ed.] London: Edward Arnold, 2000; 99-112.
4. The Management of Recurrent Miscarriage, Royal College of Obstetricians and Gynaecologists.
URL: http://www.rcog.org.uk/guidelines.asp?PageID=106&Guideline ID=46.
5. The Management of Gestational Trophoblastic Disease, Royal College of Obstetricians and Gynaecologists.
URL: http://www.rcog.org.uk/guidelines.asp?PageID=106&Guideline ID=21.
6. Hydatidiform Mole and Choriocarcinoma UK information service. URL: http://www.hmole-chorio.org.uk.
7. Nelson-Piercy C. *Handbook of Obstetric Medicine.* Oxford: Isis Medical Media, 1997; 217-226.
8. Brocklehurst P, Volmink J. Antiretrovirals for reducing the risk of mother-to-child transmission of HIV infection (Cochrane Review). In: *The Cochrane Library,* Issue 4. Oxford: Update Software, 2002.

Useful Websites

- The Miscarriage Association. This organisation has over 50 support groups across the UK. URL: http://www.the-ma.org.uk/.
- The Ectopic Pregnancy Trust. This organisation provides information and support for patients and aims to raise awareness of this disorder. URL: http://www.ectopic.org/trust/index.htm.
- The Hyperemesis Education and Research Organization. This is a US-based organisation that provides information for both clinicians and patients on this disorder. URL: http://www.hyperemesis.org/.

Problems in Later Pregnancy

Dr Arri Coomarasamy and Dr D van der Berg

Introduction

In this chapter, we concentrate on problems that can occur in pregnancy after the gestational age of viability (24 weeks). Accurate diagnosis, and timely and effective treatment of most conditions that occur in later pregnancy, can reduce the risk to the mother, baby, or both. The threshold for action tends to be lower in later pregnancy, and if in doubt, GPs should err on the side of caution and obtain advice or arrange referral sooner rather than later.

The following conditions are addressed in this chapter:
- hypertension in pregnancy
- pre-term labour
- PPROM
- IUGR
- obstetric cholestasis
- reduced/absent foetal movements
- antepartum haemorrhage
- post-term pregnancy.

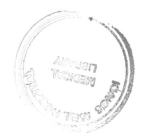

Hypertension in Pregnancy

The incidence of hypertension in pregnancy varies according to the definition used and population studied. However, most studies report an incidence of 5–10% of all pregnancies. Hypertensive disorders were the second commonest direct cause of maternal death in the most recent reports on confidential enquiries into maternal death (Scottish Executive Health Department, 1998).

Many different classifications for hypertension in pregnancy exist, making diagnosis, management, and research difficult. One commonly used classification is given below:
- chronic (pre-existing) hypertension (2% of women of child bearing age)
- pregnancy-induced hypertension without proteinuria
- pregnancy-induced hypertension with proteinuria (also called pre-eclampsia; incidence of severe pre-eclampsia is about 1% of all pregnancies).

When measuring blood pressure, it is important to use the correct procedure: the woman should be in the sitting position; arm at the level of heart; use Korotkoff phase V (disappearance) rather than IV (muffling) for diastolic pressure; use large cuffs for large arms; take at least two readings; and review the trend (more than 30mm/Hg systolic or 15mm/Hg diastolic) as well as absolute blood pressure (more than 140/90mm/Hg).

Proteinuria is substantial if urinalysis shows ≥1+ protein or there is >300mg of protein in a 24-hour collection of urine. However, urinalysis may be falsely positive in up to 25% of women with 'trace' and 6% of women with 1+ proteinuria. Therefore, consider a 24-hour urine collection for an accurate assessment of proteinuria in these women.

UTI, pre-existing renal disease, or contamination of urine with vaginal discharge can all give a positive result on urinalysis. Therefore, don't forget to send an MSU, and consider other causes of proteinuria.

Chronic (pre-existing) hypertension
This is defined as hypertension that is diagnosed before pregnancy, or that manifests in the first half (<20 weeks) of pregnancy, or persists beyond six weeks after pregnancy. This is discussed in the chapter 'Routine Antenatal and Postnatal Care'.

Pregnancy-induced hypertension without proteinuria
This appears in the second half (>20 weeks) of pregnancy and normally resolves within six weeks of delivery. This disorder complicates 5–10% of pregnancies and the outcome for the mother and foetus is as good as that for normotensive women.

The usual drug therapies used to treat hypertension in pregnancy are methyldopa (e.g. 500–3000mg/day in two to four doses) and labetalol (e.g. 200–1200mg/day in two to four doses); calcium channel blockers (e.g. nifedipine, can be given po or sublingual) are sometimes used also. However, ACE inhibitors should be avoided. Treatment guidelines often recommend non-pharmacological methods for hypertension in later pregnancy (with or without antihypertensives), especially for mildly increased blood pressure. However, there is little evidence to support non-pharmacological treatments (such as restricted activity).

Pre-eclampsia
Pre-eclampsia is a multi-system disorder characterised by hypertension and proteinuria, and generally occurs in the second half of pregnancy. The disease can present and progress in a variety of unpredictable ways. The complications that could arise from pre-eclampsia include:

Maternal:
- adult respiratory distress syndrome
- pulmonary oedema

- cerebrovascular accident
- eclampsia
- HELLP
- renal failure
- hepatic failure/rupture
- coagulation failure
- cortical blindness
- post-partum haemorrhage
- deep venous thrombosis
- fluid overload (complication of treatment).

Foetal:
- growth restriction
- placental abruption
- iatrogenic pre-term delivery.

Risk factors for pre-eclampsia
A number of risk factors exist, notably: nulliparity, age >40 years, African ethnic origin, family history of pregnancy-induced hypertension, chronic hypertension, chronic renal disease, antiphospholipid syndrome, diabetes mellitus, and multiple gestation.

Molar pregnancy, multiple pregnancy, and iso-immunisation can occasionally cause early onset of pre-eclampsia.

Diagnosis and management at primary care level
- If pre-eclampsia is suspected, obtain a full clinical history (previous or family history of hypertension or pre-eclampsia, visual symptoms, nausea and vomiting, headaches, epigastric pains, foetal movement, and medical history).
- Measure blood pressure.
- Perform urinalysis (if positive, send an MSU for culture).
- Check for hyper-reflexia and clonus.
- Measure symphyseal fundal height and listen to the foetal heart.
- FBC, urea and electrolytes, serum urate, and liver function tests are the usual initial blood tests performed but are usually best done in secondary care. Clotting is required only if severe disease is suspected or thrombocytopenia is present on FBC.
- Decide on the need for referral to secondary care (see below) and further surveillance. If in doubt, refer.
- If a day care unit is available at the local hospital, it may be possible to manage many women with mild hypertension and without proteinuria in the primary care setting, in collaboration with the day care unit.

Indications for referral for investigations and management at secondary care level
- Persistent blood pressure of >140/90mm/Hg (i.e. two or more readings).
- Blood pressure over 160/100mm/Hg needs urgent referral to hospital; if over 170/100mm/Hg, needs immediate referral to hospital (the woman will need antihypertensive treatment, regardless of cause, to protect her from CVA and MI).
- If there is any proteinuria (even trace) with hypertension.
- If the patient is unwell, refer immediately.
- If pre-eclamptic symptoms or signs are present, or any blood tests are abnormal.
- If in doubt about the need for referral, seek advice from on-call obstetrician.

Diagnosis and management at secondary care level
- Important aspects of management include an evaluation of the course of pregnancy thus far, and repeated clinical examinations, blood pressure, and urinalysis.
- Blood tests (see above) and 24-hour urine collection for protein quantification and creatinine clearance will generally be needed.
- Foetal ultrasound biometry and monitoring of foetal well-being (umbilical Doppler, CTG, and biophysical profiles) are usually performed.
- Treat severe hypertension (to protect the mother from CVA and MI, but remember that antihypertensive treatment does not stop the progression of pre-eclampsia).
- A decision on the timing and mode of delivery will be made; however, delivery does not remove the risks instantly – up to half of eclamptic fits occur postpartum.
- If pre-term delivery is anticipated, give steroid injections to improve foetal lung maturity.
- Consider magnesium sulphate for primary (in fulminating pre-eclampsia) and secondary (following convulsions) prophylaxis of eclampsia.
- Monitor fluid balance carefully.
- Management should be in close collaboration with anaesthetists, physicians, and other staff.
- Have clear guidelines for dealing with complications of pre-eclampsia (such as eclampsia, pulmonary oedema, etc).

Useful tips
- Although unlikely, how would you cope with an eclamptic fit at home?
- Call emergency help.
- Remove hard objects from around the woman so that she does not hurt herself.
- Turn her on her side and check her airway; remember ABC of resuscitation while awaiting help.
- Stop fits with intravenous, or if not possible, intramuscular injection of diazepam 10–20mg, or diazepam per rectum.
- If you do not have diazepam, use any other anticonvulsant.

Pre-term Labour and Delivery

Pre-term delivery is birth between viability (24 weeks in UK) to 37 completed weeks. The incidence is 7–11%. However, serious consequences of pre-term delivery occur before 34 weeks (incidence: 3%) and especially before 28 weeks (extreme prematurity); 70–80% of all perinatal deaths occur in pre-term infants.

Threatened pre-term labour occurs when there are persistent uterine contractions without cervical change. Actual pre-term labour occurs when the contractions are accompanied by effacement or progressive cervical dilatation. Up to 50% of women with threatened pre-term labour may not progress to delivery.

Surviving pre-term infants, especially those born at earlier gestations, may suffer serious morbidity, such as respiratory distress syndrome, intraventricular haemorrhage, necrotising enterocolitis, hypothermia, hypoglycaemia, septicaemia, persistent patent ductus arteriosus, visual impairment, hearing loss, cerebral palsy, and cognitive difficulties.

Risks to the mother include: risks from tocolytics (particularly the cardiovascular, respiratory, and endocrine side-effects of intravenous beta-agonists); operative delivery (especially, classical caesarean section – for extremely pre-term baby – is associated with increased intra-operative bleeding, infection, and compromised future uterine function); and prolonged hospitalisation (psychological morbidity).

Risk factors for pre-term labour
- Previous pre-term delivery
- PPROM
- Low socio-economic class
- Maternal age under 18 years
- Low booking BMI
- Smoking and substance abuse
- Infections (urinary tract infections, asymptomatic bacteruria, vaginal infections, and systemic infections)
- Over distension of the uterus (multiple pregnancy and polyhydramnios)
- Antepartum haemorrhage and early pregnancy bleeding
- Cervical incompetence
- Uterine abnormalities
- Foetal causes (intrauterine death, intrauterine growth restriction, congenital abnormalities)

Diagnosis and management at primary care level
- Confirm gestation (check both ultrasound and menstrual dates).
- Identify any risk or causative factors that might predispose to pre-term labour and obtain full history of the events leading up to the consultation.

- Check vitals, particularly temperature (any infection can cause pre-term labour).
- Perform urinalysis (UTI is a treatable cause of pre-term labour) and send an MSU.
- Examine abdomen to determine uterine activity; you may need to be patient for this!
- Assess foetal heart activity.
- Decide on the need for referral or further surveillance (see Useful tips below).

GPs will not normally need to perform a vaginal examination unless delivery is imminent (i.e. before transfer is possible to the nearest hospital). This is because a baseline cervical examination is likely to be performed in the hospital regardless of whether an examination in primary care was done or not.

Useful tips

○ If pre-term labour is suspected, refer to secondary care immediately.
○ Although up to 50% may not deliver pre-term, as the diagnostic tests for pre-term labour (including clinical history and examination features as well as laboratory tests) have poor accuracy, there is no reliable way of knowing who would, and who wouldn't, deliver pre-term. Given that timely effective interventions (for example, antenatal steroids and care in an intensive neonatal unit) will radically improve perinatal outcome, it is imperative to refer sooner rather than later.
○ Treatment of UTIs, asymptomatic bacteruria, and bacterial vaginosis is known to reduce the risk of pre-term delivery.

Diagnosis and management at secondary care level

- Establish gestational age and clinical history thus far.
- Assess abdomen for symphyseal fundal height, lie, presentation (USS if uncertain), engagement, and contractions or tenderness. Check for loin tenderness (indicative of pyelonephritis).
- Commence CTG (if >26 weeks)
- Pelvic examination. Try to limit to one examiner and use sterile technique. Speculum to visualise cervix, check for rupture of membranes and vaginal swab. May need digital examination to assess effacement and dilatation provided membranes are intact.
- Search for precipitating factors – urinalysis, MSU, high vaginal swab, bleeding, etc – and treat appropriately.
- Antenatal steroids, if between 24 and 36 weeks.
- Tocolysis. Only use to prolong labour by 24–48 hours to administer steroids or for in utero transfer. Ensure that there are no contraindications (chorioamnionitis, foetal death) for tocolysis.
- Ensure there is a cot in special care baby unit, and inform paediatrician (to attend delivery).

- Careful counselling by senior obstetrician and paediatricians if extreme prematurity regarding chance of survival and morbidity, mode of delivery, monitoring and management, and neonatal care.

Pre-term Pre-labour Rupture of Membranes

Pre-labour rupture of membranes occurs in 10% of all pregnancies. However, pre-term (below 37 completed weeks) rupture occurs in 2% of all pregnancies. Do not confuse these terms with prolonged rupture of membranes, which refers to rupture of membranes for more than 24 hours before delivery.

The risks of PPROM include:
- pre-term delivery – see above (over 80% deliver within seven days)
- ascending infection (incidence is 30%; however neonatal sepsis occurs in only 2–4%)
- placental abruption
- umbilical cord prolapse
- if PPROM occurs under 26 weeks, there is significant risk of pulmonary hypoplasia and various deformities
- increased incidence of retained placenta, and primary and secondary postpartum haemorrhage.

Diagnosis and management at primary care level
- Establish gestation and obtain history from the woman (how much loss, colour, any bleeding, pain, fever, rigor, foetal movements).
- Check vitals, particularly temperature.
- Palpate abdomen (for tenderness) and assess foetal heart rate (to check for foetal tachycardia).
- Observe loss on pad.
- Refer urgently to hospital if PPROM is suspected – refer immediately if ascending infection is suspected (maternal or foetal tachycardia, temperature, abdominal tenderness, etc).

Useful tips
- DO NOT DO A DIGITAL VAGINAL EXAMINATION, as this will increase the risk of ascending infection.
- The earliest clinical signs of ascending infection are foetal tachycardia and an elevation of maternal temperature (usually mild) – look out for these.

Diagnosis and management at secondary care level
As for primary care (see above), and, in addition:
- sterile speculum examination, to check for liquor and umbilical cord, and obtain a high vaginal swab

- surveillance for ascending infection – particularly assess for abdominal tenderness, temperature, foetal or maternal tachycardia, and offensive discharge – if infection is suspected, perform FBC (white cell count), C-reactive protein, MSU and blood culture, and start a broad spectrum intravenous antibiotic
- foetal surveillance, particularly with CTG and ultrasound biophysical profiles (studies show that foetal breathing movements and gross body movements cease when intra-amniotic infection develops)
- consider delivery (if there is evidence of ascending infection, foetal distress, or gestation over 34 weeks); if emergency delivery is not indicated within the first 72 hours following admission, it is safe to manage in the outpatient setting with regular monitoring for infection, foetal well-being, and growth.

If delivery is required:
- administer antenatal steroids, if between 24 and 36 weeks
- ensure there is a cot in the special care baby unit and inform paediatrician (to attend delivery).

Useful tips
How do you diagnose rupture of membranes?
○ Visualisation of amniotic fluid draining from the cervix is the most accurate test.
○ A nitrazine test may help to confirm the diagnosis. However, it should be remembered that urine, semen, and other contaminants could give a false positive result.
○ Ultrasound to diagnose reduced liquor volume in utero (due to rupture of membranes, but not necessarily so) is normally only possible with large liquor loss that would be expected to be clinically obvious. Ultrasound is, therefore, not a very useful test to diagnose rupture of membranes.
○ Regular pad checks may also help.

Intrauterine Growth Restriction

Small for gestational age refers to a foetus that has failed to achieve a specific, biometric, or weight threshold (usually below 10th, 5th, or 3rd centile) by a specific gestational age. An SGA foetus could be constitutionally small ('normal small baby') or nutritionally deprived (IUGR or, more accurately, FGR). The incidence of growth restriction varies between 3–10%, depending on the definition used and the population studied. It is the second leading cause of perinatal mortality and morbidity, following prematurity.

Growth-restricted foetuses are at increased risk of stillbirth, birth hypoxia, neonatal complications, impaired neurodevelopment, and possibly non-insulin-dependent diabetes and hypertension in adult life.

Risk factors for growth restriction include:
Maternal:
- smoking
- low socio-economic status
- pre-pregnancy weight of <50 kg
- chronic hypertension
- pre-eclampsia
- chronic renal disease
- diabetes
- collagen vascular disease
- haemaglobinopathies
- severe anaemia
- chronic pulmonary disease
- cyanotic heart disease
- recurrent antepartum haemorrhages
- drugs (steroids, beta-blockers, heroin, alcohol).

Foetal:
- chromosomal abnormalities
- genetic disorders
- congenital malformations
- in utero infections (CMV, rubella, toxoplasmosis)
- multiple gestations.

Diagnosis and management at primary care level
If the foetus is suspected to be small on abdominal palpation or on measurement of symphyseal fundal height:
- establish accurate gestation
- obtain clinical history to identify any risk factors (see above)
- refer to hospital for ultrasound biometry.

Diagnosis and management at secondary care level
- Confirm gestation.
- Arrange ultrasound biometry – if estimated foetal weight or abdominal circumference indicates a small foetus, falling growth velocity, or a reduction in liquor volume, further surveillance will be needed.
- In cases of severe growth restriction, a formal detailed scan (+ or – amniocentesis for karyotyping) and TORCH screen are needed.
- In growth-restricted foetuses, the primary surveillance tool for foetal well-being should be the umbilical artery Doppler test, as this is the only test that has been shown to reduce perinatal mortality. CTG and biophysical profiles should generally

be reserved to aid decisions on timing of delivery when the umbilical artery Doppler becomes abnormal.

- Most women with growth-restricted foetuses can be safely managed in the outpatient setting. Frequency of visit depends on severity – in most cases, twice weekly would be sufficient.

If delivery is required:
- administer steroids if gestation is below 36 weeks
- ensure paediatrician is present for delivery.

Obstetric Cholestasis

Obstetric cholestasis, also known as intrahepatic cholestasis of pregnancy, usually presents in the third trimester with pruritis (without rash) and abnormal liver enzymes. Its incidence in the UK is about 1%, although there are great geographical and racial variations. Aetiology of obstetric cholestasis is thought to be related to the cholestatic effect of circulating oestrogens.

A mother with obstetric cholestasis is at increased risk of abruptions and postpartum haemorrhage due to vitamin K deficiency, and of suffering from severe, intractable pruritis.

The foetus is at increased risk of:
- intrauterine death (often sudden and unpredictable)
- spontaneous pre-term delivery
- intracranial haemorrhage (due to vitamin K deficiency)
- intrapartum complications (meconium staining and foetal distress).

Diagnosis
The diagnosis depends on:
- history – pruritis, and rarely symptoms of biliary obstruction (pale stools, dark urine, and jaundice)
- abnormal liver function tests – particularly an increase in transaminases and bile salts
- exclusion of other causes of pruritis and abnormal liver tests:
  a. gall stones (arrange hepatobiliary tract ultrasound)
  b. viral infections (serology for hepatitis A, B, and C, cytomegalovirus, and Epstein–Barr virus)
  c. primary biliary cirrhosis and other pre-existing liver diseases (autoantibody screen).

Principles of management
- Monitor mother regularly – liver function tests, bile salts, and clotting profile.
- Monitor foetus regularly – none of the foetal monitoring tests have been shown to

predict intra-uterine death or improve outcome; however, most clinicians would use CTG and uterine Doppler test for regular monitoring of the foetus. Growth and liquor volume should be checked fortnightly.

- Treat mother's symptoms – antihistamines are sometimes used for pruritis, though some are contraindicated or caution advised in pregnancy. Consider using cholestyramine or UDCA if antihistamines are not effective.
- Give oral vitamin K to mother (10mg orally per day) from 34 weeks, especially if she has abnormal clotting, or is on cholestyramine treatment.
- Plan delivery for 38 weeks (as the foetal monitoring tests are poor predictors of sudden foetal demise, elective delivery at 38 weeks may reduce perinatal mortality associated with obstetric cholestasis).
- Give baby intramuscular vitamin K at birth.

Useful tips
○ The risks to the foetus are not proportional to the levels of liver function tests or degree of mother's symptoms.
○ UDCA improves mother's symptoms and liver function tests; however, there is no evidence to date that this translates into better outcome for the foetus.

Reduced or Absent Foetal Movements
Universal routine formal foetal movement counting is controversial – large trials show no evidence that this reduces the incidence of intrauterine death in normally formed foetuses. Moreover, it increases the frequency of other antenatal testing, admission to hospital, and elective delivery. The use of formal foetal movement counting has not been assessed in high risk pregnancies. However, foetal movement counting remains a common practice, as there is the possibility of benefit (at least to women at high risk).

The commonest method for the formal assessment of foetal movements is asking the mother to record the time taken for ten movements – if there are less than ten movements in 12 hours, further foetal assessment is recommended.

Diagnosis and management at primary care level
If pattern of movements has changed in patient's judgement that day, or there has been less than ten movements in 12 hours:
- establish gestation and obtain history (unusual distractions during the day, abdominal pain, vaginal bleeding, abdominal trauma, past obstetric and medical history)
- examine the abdomen, listen to the foetal heart and record foetal heart rate
- arrange urgent foetal surveillance in a day care unit, if available – if not, refer to the hospital; complete cessation of foetal movements warrants immediate referral.

Diagnosis and management at secondary care level
As above and:
- foetal surveillance: CTG, biophysical score, and umbilical artery Doppler have all been used, either on their own or in combination, although the best mode of foetal surveillance for reduced foetal movements is not clear
- if foetal movements remain infrequent: arrange for a foetal anomaly scan, continue foetal surveillance (no consensus on frequency of monitoring), and arrange fortnightly foetal biometry.

Antepartum Haemorrhage
Antepartum haemorrhage is defined as bleeding from the genital tract after 24 weeks of pregnancy. Incidence is 3–5% of all pregnancies. It is a leading cause of foetal and maternal morbidity and mortality. Causes of antepartum haemorrhage include:
- placenta praevia – 30% of all APH
- abruptions – 20% of all APH
- local causes (vulval or cervical infections, trauma, or tumours) – 5% of all APH
- vasa previa (bleeding of foetal origin from the vessels in the foetal membranes) – less than 1% of all APH
- bleeding disorders (such as von Willebrand's disease).

In about 40% of all women who present with APH, a firm diagnosis is not made.

Useful tips
- If shocked, institute resuscitative measures.
- Any late pregnancy bleeding, however small, needs immediate referral to the hospital. This is because much of the bleeding from an abruption, for example, can be concealed, with only a little (revealed) bleeding vaginally.
- Clinical assessment of amount of blood loss tends to be an underestimation – remember, a tennis ball size clot is approximately 500ml of blood.
- Do not do vaginal examination, as this can cause catastrophic bleeding from a placenta praevia.

The two commonest causes of APH are placenta praevia and abruptions.

Placenta praevia
Placenta praevia is defined as the insertion of placenta partially or fully in the lower segment of the uterus. There are three classification systems in common practice, although for management purposes, classification into simple 'minor' and 'major' categories is all that is required.

Minor: placenta encroaches lower segment but does not reach cervical os (Grade I), or placenta reaches cervical os but does not cover it (Grade II).

Major: placenta covers part of the cervical os (Grade III), or placenta covers the cervical os completely (even when the cervix is dilated) (Grade IV).

Risk factors for placenta praevia include:
- increasing age
- increasing parity
- previous caesarean section (incidence of placenta praevia is proportional to the number of past caesareans)
- previous abortions (both surgical and induced abortions increase the risk of placenta praevia)
- multiple pregnancy.

Risks of placenta praevia include:
- maternal death
- foetal death
- placenta acreta (abnormal adherence of placenta to the uterine wall)
- postpartum haemorrhage
- postpartum uterine infections
- surgical complications.

Diagnosis
Characteristically presents with painless bleeding. An ultrasound will accurately diagnose placenta praevia; transvaginal ultrasound has been shown to be safe, and can be employed when transabdominal ultrasound does not offer adequate views. Women who were diagnosed with low placenta on early scans should be rescanned at 34 weeks, as in many women the placenta may have moved away from the cervix with advancing gestation.

Principles of management
- Resuscitate if shocked.
- Decide whether immediate delivery is required (severe bleeding compromising mother and/or baby; advanced gestation where delaying delivery will not confer benefit) or expectant management is suitable (bleeding not severe, particularly with early gestations).

Useful tips
- If expectant management is deemed suitable, it is normally safe to manage women with placenta praevia in the outpatient setting (even for women who have experienced some bleeding).
- If there is no bleeding, there is no need to restrict normal physical activities.

○ If placenta praevia is minor (grades I and II), and foetal head is engaged (or the foetal head is below the leading edge of the placenta), aim for vaginal delivery. With major (grades III and IV) placenta praevia, caesarean section by a senior obstetrician – with suitable preparations to deal with a possible massive haemorrhage – is warranted.
○ If pre-term, don't forget steroid treatment; call paediatrician for delivery.

Placental abruptions

This is defined as bleeding from premature detachment of a normally situated placenta. The consequences of abruption depend on the amount of bleeding, part of which may be concealed and therefore difficult to quantify.

Risk factors for abruptions include:
- increasing maternal age and parity
- lower socio-economic class
- smoking
- elevated (unexplained) levels of AFP
- abdominal trauma (including external cephalic version)
- pre-eclampsia
- uterine decompression (for example, membrane rupture causing sudden release of liquor in polyhydramnios)
- prolonged rupture of membranes
- thrombophilia
- previous placental abruptions.

Risks of abruption include:
- maternal and foetal shock
- maternal and foetal mortality
- IUGR
- disseminated intravascular coagulation
- foeto–maternal haemorrhage (and possible iso-immunisation)
- postpartum haemorrhage.

Diagnosis

Abruption can present with vaginal bleeding, abdominal pain, uterine contraction, hypovolumic shock, foetal distress, or even stillbirth. The diagnosis is usually clinical. Ultrasound is not normally helpful as blood clot may have the same echo-density as placenta and, therefore, may not be easily discernable from placenta.

Principles of management

- Resuscitate if shocked.
- Decide on:
  a. immediate delivery by caesarean section (severe bleeding, foetal distress, or maternal shock)

    b. urgent vaginal delivery (mild to moderate bleeding without substantial foetal or maternal circulatory compromise)

    c. expectant management (mild bleeding; no or minimal foetal or maternal circulatory compromise; and early gestations).

- If foetus is dead, aim for vaginal delivery.
- Treat coagulopathy aggressively in collaboration with a haematologist.
- Look for and treat postpartum haemorrhage proactively.
- If pre-term, don't forget steroid treatment; call paediatrician for delivery.

Post-term Pregnancy

Post-term is defined as pregnancy exceeding 42 completed weeks (294 days or T+14) of gestation. The quoted incidence varies between 4–14%, but when a dating scan is done in the first half of the pregnancy the incidence is less than 2%. Perinatal mortality and morbidity are increased in post-term pregnancies.

Management

- Confirm gestation (from early USS report, if available).
- Do not allow pregnancies with other risk factors, such as APH, diabetes, and previous history of stillbirth, go post-term. The perinatal mortality is high.
- Offer all women with post-term pregnancy induction at 42 weeks – if declined, commence foetal surveillance (induction at 42 weeks reduces perinatal mortality).
- Several combinations of foetal surveillance methods have been assessed and are used. There is no clear evidence or consensus on which combination of tests is best but most would include measurement of amniotic fluid volume (maximum pool depth or amniotic fluid volume), biophysical profile, or CTG. (Note that umbilical Doppler is not of much value in post-term pregnancy.)
- Counsel woman carefully about the risks of continuing with pregnancy beyond term.

Further Reading

1. Kelly A, Nelson-Piercy C. *Obstetric cholestasis.* [PACE Review] London: RCOG, 2000.
2. Luckas MJM, Walkinshaw SA. *Prolonged pregnancy.* [PACE Review.] London: RCOG, 2001.
3. Duley LMM. *Tocolytic drugs for women in preterm labour* (1B). [RCOG Green-top Guideline.] October 2002.
4. Coomarasamy A, Fisk N, Gee H, Robson SC. *Investigation and management of the small for gestational age fetus (31).* [RCOG Green-top Guideline.] November 2002.
5. Scottish Executive Health Department. *Why Mothers Die.* [Report on Confidential Enquiries into Maternal Death in the United Kingdom, 1994-1996.] London: The Stationery Office, 1998.

Useful Websites

- Hypertensive disorders of pregnancy. Health Evidence Bulletins, UK, 1998. URL: http://hebw.uwcm.ac.uk/maternal/chapter2.html.
- Premature labour. Health Evidence Bulletins, UK, 1998. URL: http://hebw.uwcm.ac.uk/maternal/chapter13.html.
- Haemorrhage in late pregnancy (and labour). Health Evidence Bulletins, UK, 1997. URL: http://hebw.uwcm.ac.uk/maternal/chapter9.html.

Evidence-based Medicine in Obstetrics and Gynaecology

Dr Arri Coomarasamy

Introduction

Today, all doctors are encouraged to practice EBM, something not always easy to do as a busy GP. In this chapter, the fundamentals of EBM are discussed and some useful tools are provided to facilitate the reader in the practice of EBM.

What is Evidence-based Medicine?

Evidence-based medicine is the conscientious and judicious use of current best evidence in making decisions about the care of individual patients. The process of systematically finding, appraising, and using contemporaneous research findings as the basis of clinical decision follows four steps:

1. Formulate a structured question from a clinical problem.
2. Search the literature for any relevant article(s).
3. Evaluate (critically appraise) the article(s) for validity and usefulness.
4. Implement useful findings in clinical practice.

Formulating structured questions from clinical problems

A well-structured question is key to making the process of searching for evidence effective and efficient. Using the example of norethisterone and menorrhagia, a suggested approach employs four components:

Component	Question	Example
1. The patient or problem.	"How would I succinctly describe a group of patients?"	In women suffering with menorrhagia . . .
2. The intervention (test, treatment, process of care).	"What is the main action I am considering?"	. . . would treatment with norethisterone . . .
3. The comparison or alternative (if relevant).	"What is (are) the other option(s)?"	. . . compared with no treatment at all or other treatments . . .
4. The outcome(s) of interest.	"What do I/the patient want/not want?"	. . . lead to an improvement in their symptoms?

If you have more questions than you have time to answer, then prioritise them by importance (both to the patient and to your subsequent performance with other patients), answerability, likelihood of recurrence, and fun; and 'sell' some of them to your colleagues and teachers. Be sure to look back and evaluate each cycle of asking and answering questions, in order to learn from experience.

Searching the literature for any relevant article(s)

A key question is how do GPs (and other members of the PHCT) find relevant articles to answer their clinical question? There are several sources of information that can be used:

- EBM guidelines; e.g. RCOG guidelines, local PCT guidelines
- systematic reviews; e.g. CDSR (see below)
- primary literature; e.g. MEDLINE (see below)
- the internet (see below).

Take a hierarchical approach with your search. For example, if there is an up-to-date professional body guideline that has been developed using a systematic appraisal of available evidence that answers your specific question, then that is generally better than turning to MEDLINE to obtain the primary studies. Similarly, for therapy questions, the CDSR or other similar databases should be searched before turning to primary studies. The flowchart below represents a typical hierarchical approach for searching for evidence:

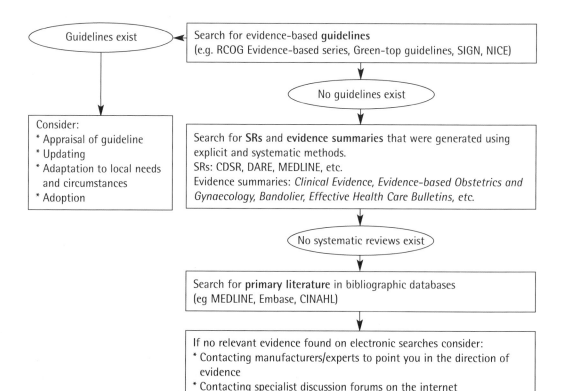

The Cochrane Database of Systematic Reviews

The CDSR contains SRs as part of the Cochrane Library, which is produced by the Cochrane Collaboration. This is an international network of individuals and institutions that prepare, maintain, and disseminate SRs of the effects of health care, and the CDSR includes the full text of the regularly updated reviews. The reviews are presented as two types: regularly updated Complete Reviews and those reviews currently under preparation, known as Protocols. Reviews are mainly of RCTs, and results are often combined statistically, with meta-analysis, to increase the power of the findings. Once a review is published it appears in every subsequent issue; reviews are revised as new research results become available or as errors are identified. The Cochrane Library is published quarterly on CD-ROM and the internet, and is distributed on a subscription basis. Some internet sites provide free access to the Cochrane Database; e.g. Doctors.net.uk (http://www.doctors.net.uk).

MEDLINE

Index Medicus, the catalogue of the United States NLM, and a periodical index to the medical literature, is available in a printed format. It is also available in electronic version, known as MEDLINE. Index Medicus is a bibliographic listing of references to articles from biomedical journals worldwide. The NLM includes articles that have been assessed as useful by a group including physicians, editors, and librarians. Trained literature analysts index selected articles and there is an annual Cumulated Index Medicus. The MEDLINE database is available from different vendors using CD-ROM technology, including Ovid Technologies (Ovid) and Silver Platter Information WinSPIRS. The MEDLINE database is the same, but the commands differ according to the software. MEDLINE can also be accessed via the internet. For example, the BMA library runs a MEDLINE service for its members, which is available 24 hours a day through the web. MEDLINE is also accessible on the web through PubMed (http://www.ncbi.nlm.nih.gov/PubMed/). This is the NLM's search service that provides access to over 11 million citations in MEDLINE, PreMEDLINE, and other related databases, as well as links to some online journals.

The internet (world wide web)

Medical research can also be found by searching the world wide web part of the internet directly. This is most easily done by using one or more of the many internet search engines such as Yahoo (http://uk.yahoo.com/), AltaVista (http://uk.altavista.com/), or Lycos (http://www.lycos.co.uk). As an alternative to these, there are a number of medical search engines. Some websites such as MEDLINE Pro (http://medlinepro.com) allow users to search a number of medical search engines in one go.

The quality of information on the web, though, is extremely variable, limiting its use as a reliable source of information. At the best of times, search engines will find only a fraction of the total literature available on the web about a particular topic, unsurprising since the number of websites continues to grow rapidly. With all search engines, the usefulness of the results will depend largely on the search strategy used, in particular the search entry term(s) used. Also, most medical information posted on the web originates from the USA, and therefore may not always be relevant to health care in other countries.

For guidance on building a search strategy, consult the following document: Searching For Evidence, Clinical Governance Advice No 3, RCOG, London UK, 2001, freely available at http://www.rcog.org.uk/mainpages.asp?PageID=318 (last visited October 2002).

Evaluating (critically appraising) the article(s) for validity and usefulness

Once you have identified and retrieved article(s) that may possibly answer your question, you need to select the good ones from the bad and the downright ugly, and this involves checking these articles for:

- validity (methodological soundness)
- importance (for example, is a *statistically* significant reduction in BP of 2mm Hg *clinically* significant?)
- applicability of the results to your patients.

Various checklists exist to help appraise different types of clinical questions. Checklists for therapeutic and diagnostic questions are given below, as examples. See 'Further reading' and 'Useful websites' at the end of the chapter for appraisal checklists for other types of clinical questions.

Appraisal checklist for therapy questions

1. Are the results valid?
- Is the assignment of patients randomised and concealed?
- Are all patients who entered the trial properly accounted and attributed for at its conclusion?
- Is follow-up complete?
- Are patients analysed in the groups to which they were randomised?
- Are patients, health workers, and study personnel 'blind' to treatment?
- Are the groups similarly at the start of the trial?
- Aside from the experimental intervention, are the groups treated equally?

2. What are the results (i.e. importance of results)?
- How large is the treatment effect? (Calculate NNT if possible, but beware that NNT changes with varying baseline risk of disease!)
- How precise is the treatment effect?

3. Will the results help me in caring for my *patients* (applicability)?
- Can the results be applied to *my* patients?
- What is the NNT for *my* patient?

○ Are all clinically important outcomes considered?
○ What are the likely benefits? Are they worth the potential harms and costs?

Appraisal checklist for diagnostic questions
1. Are the results valid?
○ Is there an independent 'blind' comparison with a reference standard?
○ Does the patient sample include an appropriate spectrum of patients to whom the test will be applied in clinical practice?
○ Do the results of the test influence the decision to perform the reference standard?
2. What are the results?
○ Are likelihood ratios, or the data necessary to calculate likelihood ratios, provided?
○ What are the likelihood ratios? What is their precision? What are the resultant post-test probabilities?
3. Will the results help me in caring for my *patients?*
○ Are the results applicable to *my* patients? What is the post-test probability in *my* patient?
○ Will the results change my management?
○ Will patients be better off as a result of the test?

Implementing useful findings in clinical practice
All too often evidence is extant and clinicians know of its findings but don't implement the care that should logically ensue. An example of this is using norethisterone to treat menorrhagia. Thus, providing the evidence, on its own, may not be enough to effect change in care.

At an individual level, evidence may be incorporated into care with your patient's consent. But this may not be all that easy, as, for example, conventions of the organisation in which you work may be against this or there may be opposing peer pressure. At an organisational level matters are much more complex. There are various tools that may aid with implementation, including:
  • education – awareness of evidence (journal clubs, publications, etc.)
  • champions/opinion leaders
  • guidelines
  • care pathways
  • audit and feedback.

As evidence-based practice aims to improve patient care – and is not just an academic exercise – careful consideration needs to be given to strategies that may improve implementation at an individual level, as well as at an organisational level.

Example: using norethisterone to treat menorrhagia

Step 1: formulating the clinical question – see above. The keywords selected for search were 'norethisterone' and 'menorrhagia'.

Step 2: searching for relevant literature. Taking a hierarchical approach, one needs to first search for evidence-based guidelines. A search on the RCOG website (www.rcog.org.uk) found the document 'National Evidence-Based Clinical Guidelines: The Initial Management of Menorrhagia', which stated, 'Low dose, luteal phase administration of norethisterone is *not* an effective treatment for menorrhagia (Grade A recommendation)'. It would therefore be legitimate to stop the search at this point, and start considering the local application of this information. However, if we assumed this guideline did not exist, then the next step would be to search for SRs and evidence summaries. A search in the Cochrane Library found there was an SR that compared luteal phase oral progestogens with danazol, tranexamic acid, and a progesterone-releasing intrauterine device (a total of seven RCTs) (Lethaby *et al*, 2002). There was a significant *increase* in mean menstrual blood loss with oral progestogens compared with the others. There were no RCTs comparing norethisterone to placebo. As a relevant and up-to-date systematic review existed, there is no reason to turn to MEDLINE in this case.

Step 3: critical appraisal. The SR used explicit and comprehensive methods, and the findings were synthesised appropriately. The primary studies in the review were themselves of good quality. We therefore can have confidence in the inferences.

Step 4: implementing useful findings in practice. Based on the clear finding of ineffectiveness of norethisterone, an individual clinician may decide to stop using this drug for treatment of menorrhagia. The RCOG guideline and the Cochrane Review could be presented in a practice journal club, with the aim of influencing local practice, alongside the RCOG guideline adapted to practice circumstances (if necessary) and adopted. The practice can then be audited to evaluate if change has been achieved.

Further Reading

1. Sackett DL, Straus SE, Richardson WS, *et al. Evidence-based Medicine: How to Practice and Teach EBM.* [2nd edition.] Edinburgh: Churchill Livingstone, 2000.
2. Greenhalgh T. *How to Read a Paper: The Basics of Evidence Based Medicine.* [2nd edition.] London: BMJ Books, 2002.
3. Haynes RB, Devereaux PJ, Guyatt GH. Physicians' and patients' choices in evidence based practice. *BMJ* 2002; **324:** 1350.
4. Godlee F. Getting evidence into practice. Needs the right resources and the right organisation. *BMJ* 1998; **317:** 6.
5. Straus SE, McAlister FA. Evidence-based medicine: a commentary on common criticisms. *CMAJ* 2000 Oct 3; **163(7):** 837-841.
6. Lethaby A, Irvine G, Cameron I. Cyclical progestogens for heavy menstrual bleeding (Cochrane review). In: *The Cochrane Library*, Issue 2. Oxford: Update Software, 2002.

Useful Websites

• Research resources: evidence-based health care, RCGP website. This provides a number of useful links to websites concerned with EBM and its application.
   URL: http://www.rcgp.org.uk/rcgp/research/resources/evidence.asp.
• For an excellent website that brings together various resources relevant to evidence-based practice, visit: 'A ScHARR Introduction to Evidence Based Practice on the Internet' at http://www.shef.ac.uk/~scharr/ir/netting/ (last visited November 2002).
• For searching for evidence, see Clinical Governance Advice No 3, RCOG, London UK, 2001, freely available at http://www.rcog.org.uk/mainpages.asp?PageID=318 (last visited October 2002).

Index

A

abortion *see* miscarriage
abruptio placentae   81
Acanthosis nigricans   102
acne
    polycystic ovarian syndrome   101
    premenstrual syndrome   2
acute pelvic vein thrombosis   82
adenomyomas, pelvic pain, chronic   89
adenomyosis   82
    dysmenorrhoea   11
    menorrhagia   4
    pelvic pain, chronic   84, 85
adhesiolysis   90
agnus castus, use in premenstrual
    syndrome   3
alcohol consumption
    foetal growth restriction, risks   151
    pre-pregnancy advice   97
    subfertility   94-5
alpha-blocking drugs, urinary
    incontinence   38
alpha fetoprotein   65, 124
amenorrhoea   13-15
    Mirena, induced by   6
    polycystic ovarian syndrome   101
    primary   13
    secondary   13-15
    when to refer?   15
amniocentesis   124-5
    karyotyping, amniotic fluid cells 124-5
anal incontinence   52-3
androgen-producing tumours,
    amenorrhoea   14

androgens
    polycystic ovarian syndrome   101-2
    postmenopausal woman   19
androstenedione, polycystic ovarian
    syndrome   101-2
anovulation   97, 99
antenatal care, general practice 15, 119-26
    antenatal surveillance   125-6
    Down's syndrome, screening   124-5
    first appointment   119-21
antenatal clinics, team work   129
Antenatal Results and Choices   129
antenatal screening, infections in
    pregnancy   139-42
antenatal steroids   148, 150, 152, 157
antenatal testing for HIV   142
antepartum haemorrhage   143, 154-7
antibiotics
    acute pelvic pain   84
    interactions with hormonal
        contraceptives   112-13
    mastitis   127
    prophylactic, coil insertion   110-11
    puerperal pyrexia   127
    secondary postpartum haemorrhage 127
    septic abortion   134
anticholinergic medications
    urinary incontinence   38, 40
        elderly patient   51-2
anticonvulsants
    fits in pre-eclampsia   146
    interactions with hormonal
        contraceptives   113
    pregnancy, teratogenic effect   124

antidepressants
    postnatal depression   128
    urinary incontinence   38
antidiuretic hormone analogues, detrusor
    overactivity, treatment   43
anti-D prophylaxis   126, 139
anti-emetics   12, 136, 138
antihistamines   43, 153
antimuscarinic drugs, urinary
    incontinence prescribing drugs   43
anti-Parkinsonian drugs, urinary
    incontinence   38
antiphospholipid syndrome,
    pre-eclampsia, risk for   145
anxiety   14, 16, 40
appendicitis   72, 82
Asherman's syndrome, amenorrhoea   14
Asian women, anaemia, pregnancy
    related   120
aspirin, low dose   27, 134
auto-antibody screen, premature
    menopause   16
autosomal trisomies   124
azoospermia   98-100, 115

B
bacterial vaginosis   10, 74-5
    pelvic pain, chronic   88
    pregnancy   138-9
benzodiazepines
    dependency   3
    premenstrual syndrome   3
    urinary incontinence   38
beta-blockers, foetal growth restriction,
    risks   151
b-hCG   124
    hydatiform moles   137
bisphosphonates   29-30
    osteoporosis, prevention   31
black cohosh   30
bladder   36
    female, drill   44

female, what's normal?   41
painful   49-50
tumours   37
blighted ovum   131
blood pressure monitoring
    pregnancy   121-2, 144
    while on pill   109
body mass index
    low, risk for pre-term labour and
      delivery   147
    pill, contraindication for   107-8
body temperature (basal), menstrual
    cycle   2
bone
    density   21
      pregnancy   111
      screening   28
    loss, menopause, hormone
      replacement treatment   21
    mass, osteoporosis, WHO
      definition   30
BRCA-1 gene mutation   64
breast cancer
    detection, well woman clinics   31
    hormone replacement therapy
      associated with   21-4
      relative contraindication   26
    screening   57
breast engorgement   127
breast feeding
    baby's immune system   139
    infections, transmission   139
    ovarian cancer, protective effect
      against   64
    problems   126-7
breast milk   126
breast self-examination instructions   31
brush smear, cervical smear   58-9

C
CA125   65
CA19.9   65

caesarean section
  herpes simplex virus infection,
    transmission prevention   77
  placental abruption   156
caesarean sections, risks associated   147
calcitonin   31
calcitriol   31
calcium   3, 30-1
  diet, osteoporosis prevention   31
calcium antagonists, urinary
  incontinence   38
calcium channel blocking drugs, urinary
  incontinence, elderly patient   51-2
candida infection   58, 75
  pregnancy   138-9
cardiotocography   150, 151-4
cerebrovascular accidents, hormone
  replacement therapy, associated
    with   23-4
cervical cancer
  detection, well woman clinics   31
  screening   57-62
    abnormal, management   61-2
    NHS programme   58
    pre-malignant disease   57-8
    results   60-1
cervical caps   107
cervical ectopy   10
cervical incompetence, pre-term delivery,
  risk for   147
cervical screening, prior to hormone
  replacement therapy   28
cervical smear
  abnormal   10
    referral to a gynaecologist   6
  dysfunctional uterine bleeding   8
  well women clinics   32
cervix, incompetence   132, 134
chemotherapy
  amenorrhoea   14
  ovarian cancer   66
  premature menopause   16

  vulval cancer   67
chickenpox, in pregnancy   139-40
Chlamydia trachomatis infection   10, 58,
  69-74, 89, 94, 96, 141
Cholestasis   126, 143
chromosomal abnormalities   131-3
CIN grades
  cervical smear   57-8
    risk factors for   58
  human papillomavirus   77
climacteric phase *see* perimenopause
clomiphene   99
  ovulation induction   97
  polycystic ovarian syndrome   104
clotrimazole   76
  pregnancy   139
coeliac disease, pelvic pain, chronic   84
coil *see also* intrauterine contraceptive
  device   113-14
coital frequency/timing   94
collagen vascular disease, foetal growth
  restriction, risks   151
colorectal cancer   64
colposcopy
  abnormal cervical smear   61-2
colposuspension   49
combined oral contraceptive pill   107-110
  after molar pregnancy   137
  amenorrhoea   14
  contraindications   108-9
  dysfunctional uterine bleeding   9
  dysmenorrhoea   12
  endometriosis   92
  essential information before the first
    prescription   107-8
  irregular bleeding   9
  menorrhagia   7(fig.)
  monitoring   109
  ovarian cancer, protective effect
    against   64
  pelvic pain, chronic   89-90
  premenstrual syndrome   3

progestogen-only pill –
  the mini-pill   106, 109-10
  side-effects   109
  venous thromboembolism, risk of   107
  which pill?   109
complete miscarriage   133
condoms   106
  sexually transmitted infection
    transmission, prevention   73
congenital rubella syndrome   140
congenital syphilis syndrome   140-1
congenital toxoplasmosis   141
Conn's syndrome, pregnancy, pre-existing
  maternal medical problems   121
continence advisers   50-1
contraception (see also family planning)
  emergency see emergency
    contraception
  failure rates   105-6
  hormonal, drug interactions   112-13
  natural methods   114
  NHS prescriptions   105
  post-coital (hormonal), nurse
    issuing   110, 118
  unprotected sexual
    intercourse   110-11, 118
  while on hormone replacement
    therapy   29
cordocentesis, acquired toxoplasmosis
  during pregnancy   141
corpus luteum   2
  cyst, rupture   81
corticosteroids, bone loss   30
counselling
  amenorrhoea   14
  breast feeding   127
  Depo-Provera   111
  Down's syndrome   124-5
  ectopic pregnancy
    methotrexate intratubal
      injection   135
    while on pill   110

female sterilisation   116
genetic, ovarian cancer   64-5
herpes simplex virus infection   77
hormone replacement therapy   27
infertility, regarding adoption   100
loss of pregnancy   139
menopause   31-2
missed miscarriage   133
pelvic pain, chronic   90
pregnancy, consanguineous
  relationship   119
premenstrual syndrome   3
pre-pregnancy, anticonvulsant
  drugs, use   124
pre-term labour   149
vasectomy   115
cryocautery   61
Cushing's syndrome, pregnancy,
  pre-existing maternal medical
    problems   121
cyclic vulvovaginitis, medical treatment 92
cystic fibrosis screen   98
cystocele   53
cytomegalovirus   140, 152
  breast milk transmission   139
cystourethroscopy, pelvic pain, chronic   89

D
day care unit, mild hypertension in
  pregnancy   145
deep venous thrombosis   145
delivery (see also labour)
  at home, by midwife   121
  mode of, decision in pre-eclampsia 146
  pre-term   147-9
Depo Provera   3, 8, 12, 14, 58, 111-12
depression   2, 20, 27, 51
detrusor   36
  activity   41
  contraction, failure, voiding
    difficulties   49
  instability   40-1

overactivity 40-1
  treatment 41-5, 48
detrusor hyperreflexia 36
detrusor sphincter dyssynergia 49
diabetes mellitus 27, 40, 51, 101, 103, 122-3, 132, 145, 151
diaphragms 106
diet
  gestational diabetes in pregnancy 123
  premenstrual syndrome 3-4
dihydroepiandrosterone sulfate (DHEAS) 15
disc herniation, pelvic pain, chronic 85
disseminated intravascular coagulation,
  septic abortion 134
diuretics 3, 38, 51
diverticular disease
  barium enema 89
  pelvic pain, chronic 84
Down's syndrome
  screening 124-5
    antenatal care, first visit 120
doxazosin, urinary incontinence 38
doxycycline 71-2, 73
dual energy X-ray absorptiometry (DEXA) 30
dye test, infertility 98
dyschezia 81
dysesthetic vulvodynia, medical treatment 92
dysfunctional uterine bleeding 4, 8-9
dyskaryosis 60-2, 77
dysmenorrhoea 11-13, 81
  Mirena, treatment in 6
  pelvic pain, chronic 84-5
dyspareunia 81
  deep 85
  dysmenorrhoea, secondary 11
  menopause 20
  pelvic pain, chronic 85
  post-coital ache with 85
  psychosexual counselling 91
dysuria 37

E
early pregnancy assessment unit 133
eclampsia 122, 145
ectopic pregnancy 134-5
  acute pelvic pain, pregnancy related 81-3
  diagnosis 134-5
  investigations 135
  laparoscopy 83
  management 135
  pelvic inflammatory disease 69
  pelvic inflammatory disease, versus 72
  risk while on pill 110
  shocked patient, resuscitation 135
ejaculatory difficulty 95
elderly patient (women), incontinence 50-1
emergency contraception 110-11
endocervical glandular lesion (AIS or CGIN) 59
endo-cervical swab 73
endometrial balloon, menorrhagia 8
endometrial biopsy, amenorrhoea 15
endometrial cancer 8, 62-4
  hormone replacement therapy associated with 21, 23
    relative contraindication 26
endometrial hyperplasia 8, 63
  menorrhagia 4
  polycystic ovarian syndrome 102, 103
endometrial sampling
  endometrial cancer, suspected 63
  menorrhagia 5
endometriosis 82
  analgesia 89-90
  dysmenorrhoea 11
  dyspareunia, deep 85
  hormone replacement therapy, contraindication 27
  infertility 100
  laparoscopy 12
  treatment 100

medical treatment 92
menorrhagia 8
pelvic pain, chronic 84, 85
rectovaginal examination 88
uterosacral ligament palpation 88
enterocele 53
epidural anaesthesia, acute urinary
retention 48
epilepsy, pre-existing maternal medical
problem 124
epithelial ovarian cancer, hormone
replacement therapy, associated with 23
Epstein-Barr virus 152
erectile difficulty 95
evacuation of retained products of
conception 127, 132-4
evidence-based medicine 159-65
literature searching 160-2
evaluating (critically
appraising) 162-3
implementing findings in clinical
practice 163
exercise 3, 14, 30, 97, 102

F
faecal impaction, elderly women,
incontinence 51
family planning 58, 105-16
female sterilisation 114-16
failure rate 116
positive pregnancy test 139
postpartum 115
regretting after 115
fertility, factors adversely affecting 94
fibroids 4, 81, 85
fibromyalgia 84
fistulae, incontinence from 50
fits, eclamptic, postpartum 146
Fitz-Hugh-Curtis syndrome 72
fluid overload 145
fluid retention, premenstrual
syndrome 3

fluoxetine, use in premenstrual
syndrome 3
foetal distress 152-3
foetal growth restriction 122
foetal movements, reduced/absent
143, 153-4
foetal surveillance
obstetric cholestasis 152-3
pre-term pre-labour rupture of
membranes 150
foetal varicella syndrome 139
folic acid
diabetes in pregnancy 122
during pregnancy 121
preconceptually, women taking
anticonvulsants 124
pre-pregnancy advice 97
prior to conception 121
follicle-stimulating hormone
menopause 19-20
premature 15-16
menstrual cycle, luteal phase 2
polycystic ovarian syndrome 101
prior to hormone replacement
therapy 28
subfertility, initial investigations 95
frequency in pregnancy 138
full blood count 5, 8,
16, 32, 83, 89, 95, 120, 150

G
galactorrhoea 14, 94
gall stones, pregnancy 152
Gardnerella infection 59, 74
genital swabs 10, 73, 76-7, 89
genuine stress incontinence 36
genuine stress incontinence, treatment
45-8
biofeedback 46
conservative measures 45
devices to aid continence 46-7
oestrogen 46

perineometry   46
physiotherapy   45-6
surgery   47-8
gestational age of viability   132
gestational diabetes mellitus   122-3
    risk factors associated with   123
    treatments   123
gestational trophoblastic disease   137
Gillick competence   118
glandular neoplasia, cervical smear   60-1
glycosuria, pregnancy-induced
    diabetes   123, 126
GnRH analogues   4, 90
gonadotrophin levels, premature
    menopause   15-16
gonorrhoea   71, 89, 141

H
H₂ antagonists, sperm count reduction   96
haematosalpinx, ectopic pregnancy   135
haematuria, macroscopic   37
haemaglobinopathies, foetal growth
    restriction, risks   151
haemoglobin, levels, menorrhagia   5
HbA1c levels, diabetes in pregnancy   122
hCG   65
headache in pregnancy   138
heavy periods see menorrhagia
HELLP syndrome   145
heparin   134
hepatitis A/B/C viruses   152
hepatitis B
    immunoglobulin   142
    screening, antenatal care, first visit 120
    transmission, prevention   73, 141-2
    vaccine   142
herbal medicines   32
    alternatives to hormone replacement
        therapy   30
    dysmenorrhoea   12
hereditary non-polyposis colorectal
    cancer   64

heroin, foetal growth restriction,
    risks   151
herpes simplex virus infection   77, 141
herpes zoster, pelvic pain, chronic   85
hip fractures, hormone replacement
    therapy, associated with   24
hirsutism
    cosmetic measures   103
    polycystic ovarian syndrome   101
HIV infection   72
    breast milk transmission   139
    delivery   142
    transmission, prevention   73
hormonal imbalance, amenorrhoea   14
hormone replacement therapy
    after molar pregnancy   137
    alternatives   29-30
    benefits   21
    contraception   29
    contraindications   26-7
    counselling   27
    endometrial cancer   63
    monitoring   28
        well woman clinics   31
    osteoporosis, prevention   31
    practical prescribing   23-9
    premature menopause   16
    risks associated with its use   21-3
        aims of therapy   21
        disorders associated with   22-3
        symptoms associated with   22
    types
        oestrogens   24-5
        period-free   26
        progestogens   25
        three-monthly bleed   26
hot flushes   20
human papillomavirus   58, 62, 77
hydatiform moles   137
hydrosalpinx   72
hymen, imperforate   13
hyperemesis gravidarum   136-7

hyperprolactinaemia 95
hypertension
  family history, hormone replacement
    therapy, contraindication 27
  pregnancy related 143-6
    chronic (pre-existing) 144
    classification 143
    incidence 143
    pre-eclampsia 144-6
    pre-existing maternal medical
      problems 121-2
    pregnancy-induced without
      proteinuria 144
hypoadrenalism, premature menopause 16
hypoparathyroidism, premature
  menopause 16
hypothalamic-pituitary-gonadal-uterine
  interaction 13-14
hypothyroidism 4, 10, 132
hysterectomy (see also total abdominal
  hysterectomy)
  bilateral salpingoophorectomy,
    last resort 4
  endometrial cancer 63
  menorrhagia, lifetime risk 4
  ovaries conserved, early
    menopause 19
  pelvic clearance 73
  subcutaneous oestrogen implants 24-5
hysterocontrastsonography 98
hysterosalpingography 98
hysteroscopy 5, 11, 63, 98

I
imipramine 50
  incontinent elderly patient 52
immunodeficiency, CIN, risk factor for 58
immunoglobulins, transplacental 139
impaired glucose tolerance 123
implants 112
incomplete miscarriage 132-3
incontinent patient 50-2

inevitable miscarriage 132
infertility 93-104
  causes 93
  factors adversely affecting
    fertility 94
  history, key points 94-7
  investigations 95-6
    secondary care 98-9
  pelvic inflammatory disease 69
  polycystic ovarian syndrome 100-4
  premature menopause 16
  pre-pregnancy advice 97
  seminal fluid analysis 96
  treatment 97-100
  unexplained 100
inflammatory bowel disease 82
  barium enema 89
inhibin-A (inhibin) 124
insulin
  polycystic ovarian syndrome 102
  requirements in pregnancy 122-3
intermenstrual bleeding
  causes 9-10
  cervical cancer 62
  diagnosis 10
  hysteroscopy 5
  investigations 10
  management 10-11
  menorrhagia 6
  referral to gynaecologist 10
internet 161-2
interstitial cystitis 49
  dyspareunia, deep 85
  pelvic pain, chronic 84
intrahepatic cholestasis of
  pregnancy 152-3
intrauterine contraceptive device 7, 11, 12, 110-11
  'lost' 94
  pelvic inflammatory disease, risk
    factor 69
  positive pregnancy test 139

progestogen-releasing   7(fig.)
intrauterine growth restriction   124,
                                126, 143, 150-2
intrauterine insemination   99-100
intravaginal ring, oestrogen   25
intravenous fluid rehydration, hyperemesis
     gravidarum   136
in utero infection, foetal growth
     restriction, risks   151
in vitro fertilisation   99
iron deficiency anaemia   5
iron therapy, oral   9
irritable bowel syndrome 12, 84, 85, 90, 92
iso-immunisation, pre-eclampsia,
     risk for   145

K
karyotype   98
karyotyping   13, 15
     premature menopause   16
knife cone biopsy   61

L
labour, pre-term   147-9
labour *see also* delivery
lactation   126-7
     amenorrhoea   14
     contraceptive protection   126
     suppression   127
lactobacillus recolonisation   76
laparoscopy
     dysmenorrhoea, resistant   12
     ectopic pregnancy, diagnosis   83, 135
     endometriosis   12
     female sterilisation   115
     pelvic inflammatory disease   71
          diagnosis   72
     pelvic pain
          acute   83-4
          chronic   89-90
     tubal patency, infertility   98
large-for-dates uterus   126

large loop excision of transformation
     zone (LLETZ)   61
laser vapourisation   61
latex, allergic reactions   106
leiomyomas, pelvic pain, chronic   84, 89
Levonelle-2   110-11
levonorgestrel   22, 109
     intrauterine system   3-4, 6, 9,
                                     12, 14, 112
libido   20, 25
liquid-based cytology   61-2
low abdominal pain, dysmenorrhoea   11-12
low back pain, pelvic pain, chronic   84
lower urinary tract, innervation   36
luteinising hormone
     amenorrhoea   14
     menopause   19-20
     menstrual cycle   1
          luteal phase   2
     polycystic ovarian syndrome   101
     subfertility, initial investigations 95-6

M
macrosomia   123
     risk of   126
magnesium sulphate, pre-eclampsia,
     fulminating   146
malpresentation (after 36 weeks)   126
mammography, prior to hormone
     replacement therapy   28
mastitis   127
maternal death, hypertensive
     disorders   143
maternity benefits   121
meconium staining   152
medroxyprogesterone acetate   3, 8,
                                    12, 22, 90, 92
mefenamic acid   9, 12-13, 89-90
     menstrual loss, reduction   5, 7(fig.)
menarche   1
menopause   1
     artificial/surgical   19

bone loss   21
cardiovascular risk   21
colon cancer   21
definition   19
diagnosis   20
early, osteoporosis risk   30
endocrinology   19-20
hormonal changes   19
HRT see hormone replacement
    therapy
natural   19
perimenopause, management   20
physiology   19-20
premature   15-16
    amenorrhoea   14
    surgical   15-16
senile dementia   21
urinary incontinence   37
menorrhagia   1, 4-8
blood loss, excessive   4
causes   4
dysmenorrhoea, secondary   11
investigations   5
medical management   5, 7(fig.)
morbidity associated   5
treatment   5-8
menstruation
abnormalities   1-17
absence see amenorrhoea
calendar   8
cycle   1-2
irregularities, polycystic ovarian
    syndrome   102
missed or delayed, causes   14
mesenteric adenitis   82
methotrexate, intratubal injection,
    ectopic pregnancy   135
migraine
family history, hormone replacement
    therapy, contraindication   27
pill, contraindication for   108-9
mini-pill   109-10

Mirena   3-4, 6, 112
amenorrhoea   112
menorrhagia   6, 112
use in
    dysmenorrhoea   6
    polycystic ovarian syndrome   102
    premenstrual syndrome   6
miscarriage   131-4
acute pelvic pain, pregnancy
    related   81, 83
Depo Provera, after   111
polycystic ovarian syndrome   101
missed miscarriage   133
mittelschmerz   81
mixed incontinence   48
molar pregnancy   136, 137
pre-eclampsia, risk for   145
registration   137
ultrasound   136
monoclonal Ab tests for b-hCG   135
ectopic pregnancy, normal
    pregnancy   135
morning sickness   138
mother-to-be, dietary advice   121
multiple sclerosis, urinary
    incontinence   40
mumps, infertility   94
myeloma, urinary incontinence   40
myofascial pain syndromes   91
pelvic pain, chronic   84, 86

N

nausea, pregnancy related see hyperemesis
    gravidarum
Neisseria gonorrhoeae   69-71
neonatal hyperbilirubinaemia   123
neonatal hypoglycaemia   123
neonatal tetanus   139
nephrolithiasis   82
neural tube defect   124
neuroablative procedures   91
neurogenic detrusor overactivity   36

nitrazine paper, amniotic fluid
  detection   139, 150
nocturia   37, 39
  incontinent elderly patient   51-2
non-steroidal anti-inflammatory drugs
  dysmenorrhoea   12
  endometriosis   89-90, 92
  menstrual loss, reduction   5
norethisterone   5, 6, 9, 22, 25, 109
nuchal translucency   125
nucleic acid amplification tests   73

O

obesity
  laparoscopy in ectopic pregnancy   135
  polycystic ovarian syndrome   101
  urinary incontinence   37
obstetric cholestasis   143, 152-3
oestradiol   24-5
  corpus luteum secretion   2
  menstrual cycle   1
  premature menopause   15-16
oestrogen
  depletion, bone loss   21
  detrusor overactivity, treatment   42
  intermenstrual bleeding   9
  menopause   16, 19-20
  menstrual cycle   1
  premenstrual syndrome   2
  relation to nausea and vomiting   136
  urinary incontinence   40, 46
oestrogen receptor modulators   31
oestrogen(s), hormone replacement
  therapy administration, routes   24-6
oestrogens, obstetric cholestasis   152
oligoasthenoteratozoospermia   98
oligohydramnios   126
oligomenorrhoea
  polycystic ovarian syndrome   102
  subfertility   95-6
oligospermia   98
omentectomy   66

oocyte donation   99
  premature menopause   16
oophorectomy, ovarian cancer   66
oral glucose tolerance tests   123
osteoporosis
  definition, WHO   30
  Depo Provera   111
  fractures, morbidity and mortality   30
  menopause   16
  pelvic pain, chronic   84
  polycystic ovarian syndrome   103
  prevention   31
  prophylaxis   29
  treatment   31, 33
ovarian cancer   64-6
  genetic counselling   64-5
  hormone replacement therapy,
    relative contraindication   26
  late presentation   64
  management   66
  protective effects against   64
  risk factors   64
  transvaginal ultrasound scan   65
  tumour markers   65
ovarian cyst
  accident   81
  recurrent, medical treatment   92
ovarian diathermy   99
ovarian/internal iliac varices,
  transcatheter embolotherapy   91
ovarian neoplasm, polycystic ovarian
  syndrome   103-4
ovulation   1, 96
ovum   2

P

pad test   41
pain clinics   91
painful periods _see_ dysmenorrhoea
pain nurse   91
pain psychologist   91
parvovirus B19   140

pelvic abscess 72
pelvic adhesions, dyspareunia, deep 85
pelvic congestion syndrome 90, 92
pelvic floor
    exercises 40, 54
    strength, examination 38
pelvic floor muscles 45
pelvic floor tension myalgia 86
    medical treatment 91-2
pelvic inflammatory disease 69-74
    acute, risk factors 69-70
    diagnosis 71
    dysmenorrhoea 11
    examination findings 70-1
    incidence 69
    menorrhagia 4
    pelvic pain, chronic 84
    prevention 73-4
    secondary care 72-3
    symptoms and signs 70
    treatment 71-2
    tubal damage, permanent 69
    when to refer? 72
pelvic neoplasm 82
pelvic organ prolapse 53-5
    pessaries 54
pelvic pain 81-92
    acute 81-3
    chronic 84-91
pelvic thrombophlebitis 127
pelvic ultrasound
    dysfunctional uterine bleeding 8
    menorrhagia 5
    pelvic inflammatory disease 72
    pelvic pain
        acute 83
        chronic 89
    prior to hormone replacement
        therapy 28
peppermint oil 90
percutaneous epididymal sperm
    aspiration 100

perimenopause 19-20
perinatal infections 141-2
perineal hygiene 39
perineometry 46
period-free hormone replacement
    treatment 22, 26
pessaries 54
    oestrogen 46
phaeochromocytoma, pregnancy, pre-
    existing maternal medical problems 121
phasic pills 109
phyto-oestrogens 30, 32
pill see combined oral contraceptive pill
pituitary tumour, amenorrhoea 14, 15
placenta acreta 155
placental abruption 122, 126, 156-7
placenta praevia 126, 154-6
polycystic ovarian syndrome 100-4
    amenorrhoea, cause of 96
    androgen excess 101-2
    bleeding, anovulatory women 8
    hirsutism 102-3
    obesity 103
    oral contraceptive pill, benefits 102
    ovulation restoration, metformin in
        overweight women 99
    subfertility 102
    weight reduction, calorie restriction
        diet 97
polyhydramnios 126
post-coital bleeding 11, 62
post-coital contraception 110-11
postnatal care in GP 126-9
postnatal depression 127-8
postnatal psychosis 128
post-partum haemorrhage 145
'post-pill amenorrhoea' 14
pre-eclampsia 144-6
    foetal growth restriction, risks 151
    placental abruption, risk for 156
    review 122, 126
pregnancy

amenorrhoea, secondary 14-15
antenatal care by GP 119-26
   low-risk, first hospital
      attendance 119
   candidiasis 75
   cornual 135
   diabetic control during 122-3
   early, problems 131-42
   folic acid prior to conception
      and during 121
   herpes simplex virus infection 77
   hypertension in see hypertension
   induced hypertension 122
   infections 139-42
   later, problems 143-58
   minor disorders 137-9
   occurring with coil 114
   ovarian cancer, protective
      effect against 64
   post-term 143, 157
   relaxation classes by midwives 121
   wanted, loss see miscarriage
pregnancy test, urinary
   amenorrhoea 14
   uterine/tubal pregnancy ruptured 82-3
premature ovarian failure 15-16
premenstrual syndrome 2-4
presacral neurectomy 13, 91
pre-term infants, morbidity 147
pre-term pre-labour rupture of
   membranes 147, 149-50
primary antiphospholipid syndrome 134
primary biliary cirrhosis 152
progesterone
   cervical smear, effect on 59
   corpus luteum secretion 2
   menopause 19
   menstrual cycle 1
   polycystic ovarian syndrome 101
   premenstrual syndrome 2
   subfertility, initial investigations 95-6
progestogen-only pill 10, 109-10

progestogen-releasing intrauterine
   system 25
progestogens
   hormone replacement therapy
      administration, routes 25-6
   menorrhagia 6
   pelvic pain, chronic 90
   premenstrual syndrome 3
prolactin
   elevated, pituitary fossa MRI 98
   polycystic ovarian syndrome 101-2
   subfertility, initial investigations 95-6
prolactinoma 95
propiverine, detrusor overactivity,
   treatment 42
prostaglandins 11
proteinuria 143-4
   pre-eclampsia 144-6
pruritus, pregnancy 152-3
puberty, delayed 13
puerperal pyrexia 127
puerperium 126
pulmonary oedema 144
punch biopsy 61
pyometra 63
pyosalpinx 72

R
radical vulvectomy 67
radiotherapy
   amenorrhoea 14
   premature menopause 16
raloxifene 31
reconstructive tubal surgery, success
   rates 99
rectocele 53
recurrent miscarriage 133-4
resuscitation, obstetric haemorrhage 154-6
rubella 140
rubella immunity 95
   antenatal care, first visit 120
   pre-pregnancy advice 97

S

sacrospinous fixation/colpopexy   55
salpingectomy, ectopic pregnancy   135
salpingitis, chronic   72
secondary postpartum haemorrhage   127
selective oestrogen receptor
    modulators   29
self-catheterisation, intermittent   50-1
seminal fluid analysis   95
sensory urgency   36, 49
septic abortion   134
septic shock   82
serotonin
    depression   2
    premenstrual syndrome   2
sex hormone binding globulin   102-3
sexual abuse   82
sexually transmitted diseases
    condoms, protection against   106
    maternal prevention in pregnancy   141
    procaine benzylpenicillin   141
    transmission, prevention   73
    viruses   62
shared care in pregnancy   119, 128
sickle cell disease, pill,
    contraindication for   108
skull X-ray, amenorrhoea   15
small-for-dates uterus   126
smoking
    CIN, risk factor for   58
    foetal growth restriction, risks   151
    infertility   94-5
    osteoporosis, fractures   30-1
    placental abruption, risk for   156
    pre-pregnancy advice   97
    pre-term delivery, risk for   147
    urinary incontinence   37
sperm dysfunction   95, 99-100
    treatment   99-100
spermicide, allergic reactions   106
spina bifida   121
    folic acid supplements   121

spinal analgesia, acute urinary
    retention   48
spine neoplasm, pelvic pain, chronic   85
spironolactone   103
    sperm count reduction   96
spontaneous miscarriage   131-4
Staphylococcus aureus mastitis   127
sterilisation, male and female   114-16
steroid injections, foetal lung
    maturity   146, 152
steroids, anabolic   95
steroids, foetal growth restriction, risks 151
stress incontinence   36
stress, reduction
    exercise   3
    irritable bowel syndrome   90
    premenstrual syndrome   3
subcutaneous oestrogen implants   24-5
subfertility   93-104
    polycystic ovarian syndrome   101
suprasacral cord lesion   49
syphilis   140-1

T

tachyphylaxis   25
    oestrogen implants   25
tampon   1, 47, 71
tension-free vaginal tape   48
termination of pregnancy   15
    Depo Provera, after   111
    hyperemesis gravidarum   137
    molar pregnancy   137
    pelvic inflammatory disease,
        risk factor   69
testicular feminisation   13
testicular sperm aspiration   100
testosterone
    amenorrhoea   15
    implant   25
    polycystic ovarian syndrome   101
    subfertility, initial investigations   95
ThinPrep Pap Test   62

threatened miscarriage   132
thrombophilia
   pill, contraindication for   107-8
   placental abruption, risk for   156
   screen   27-8
thrombophilic defects   134
thyroid disorders, amenorrhoea   14
thyroid function tests
   dysfunctional uterine bleeding   8
   intermenstrual bleeding   10
   menorrhagia   5
   prior to hormone replacement
     therapy   28
   thyrotoxicosis   136
tibolone   29
tocolytics, risks from   147-8
tolterodine   42, 50
TORCH screen   151
total abdominal hysterectomy   66
toxic shock syndrome   71
toxoplasma   141
tranexamic acid   5, 7(fig.)
   dysfunctional uterine bleeding   9
transcervical resection of the
   endometrium, menorrhagia   8
transcutaneous electrical nerve
   stimulation   12
transvaginal ultrasound
   endometrial cancer, suspected   63
   ovarian cancer   65;
   placenta previa   155
   polycystic ovarian syndrome   100
travel sickness   136
Trichomonas infection   59
tri-cyclic antidepressants, detrusor
   overactivity, treatment   43
trophoblastic disease, pregnancy, pre-
   existing maternal medical problems   121
trospium chloride, detrusor overactivity,
   treatment   43
tubal damage, pelvic inflammatory
  disease   69

tubal infertility, treatment   99
tubo-ovarian abscess   72
tumour markers, ovarian cancer   65
Turner's syndrome   13, 16

U
ulcerative colitis, pelvic pain, chronic   86
ultrasound
   acquired toxoplasmosis during
   pregnancy   141
   early pregnancy   132
   'empty uterus'   139
   foetal varicella syndrome   139
   hydatiform moles   137
ultrasound foetal biometry   122, 146
umbilical artery Doppler   151, 154
umbilical cord prolapse   149
unprotected sexual intercourse,
   emergency contraception   110-11
urethral syndrome   86
   pelvic pain, chronic   84
   urinary incontinence   40
urethritis, dyspareunia, deep   85
urgency   37, 39
   causes   40
urgency-frequency syndrome   49
urge urinary incontinence   36
urinalysis
   acute pelvic pain   83
   antenatal care, first visit   120
   pelvic pain, chronic   89
   proteinuria, pregnancy   144
   superimposed pre-eclampsia,
     screening for   122
   urinary tract infection, elimination   38
urinary diversion   51
urinary incontinence   35-45
   behavioural therapy   44
   biofeedback   44
   bladder drill   44
   definition   35
   detrusor overactivity, treatment   41-5

drugs affecting   38
examination   38
frequency/volume chart   39
history, taking   36-7
hypnotherapy   44-5
investigations   38-40
menopause   20
prevalence   35
quality of life   38
risk factors   37
symptoms   37
teams, multidisciplinary   40
terminology   36
when to refer and why?   40
urinary retention, acute/chronic   48-9
urinary tract infection   82
  elderly woman, incontinence   51
  pre-term labour, risk for   147
  recurrent, pregnancy-induced   126
  urinary incontinence, elimination in   38
urodynamic diagnosis   40-1
urodynamic stress incontinence   36-7
uroflowmetry voiding   41
urolithiasis, pelvic pain, chronic   84
ursodeoxycholic acid   153
uterine nerve ablation   13
uterine prolapse   53
uterine retroversion   85, 92
uterine rupture   81

V
vaginal cancer   66-7
vaginal cones   45-6
vaginal dilators   92
vaginal discharge
  cervical cancer   62
  cervical smear   58-60
  herpes simplex virus infection   77
  pregnancy   138-9
  vulvovaginal infections   74-8

vaginal dryness, menopause   20
vaginal oestrogens   25
vaginismus   88, 92
varicella zoster immunoglobulin
  therapy   140
varicocele   98
vasa previa   154
vasectomy   114-15
vault prolapse   53, 55
venereal infection   94
venous thromboembolism
  family history, hormone replacement
    therapy, contraindication   27
  hormone replacement therapy,
    associated with   23-4
  risk for women on pill   107, 109
vesicovaginal fistulae   50
vitamin B6   3, 136
vitamin C   3
vitamin D   30
  supplements   31
vitamin E   3
vitamin K
  deficiency   152
  intramuscular, to baby at birth   153
  oral, obstetric cholestasis   153
vitamins, supplements   3
voiding difficulties   48-9
vulval cancer   66-7
vulval herpes   48
vulval preinvasive and invasive
  disease   66-7
vulvar vestibulitis, medical treatment   92
vulvovaginal infections   74-8

W
well woman clinics   31-2
'whiff test'   74
Willebrand's disease   154
withdrawal bleed   22